WORK, HEALTH AND WELLBEING

The challenges of managing health at work

Edited by Sarah Vickerstaff, Chris Phillipson and Ross Wilkie

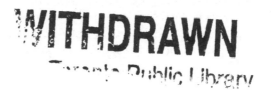

First published in Great Britain in 2013 by

The Policy Press
University of Bristol
Fourth Floor
Beacon House
Queen's Road
Bristol BS8 1QU
UK
t: +44 (0)117 331 4054
f: +44 (0)117 331 4093
tpp-info@bristol.ac.uk
www.policypress.co.uk

The Policy Press
c/o The University of Chicago Press
1427 East 60th Street
Chicago, IL 60637, USA
t: +1 773 702 7700
f: +1 773-702-9756
sales@press.uchicago.edu
www.press.uchicago.edu

British Library Cataloguing in Publication Data
A catalogue record for this book is available from the British Library.

Library of Congress Cataloging-in-Publication Data
A catalog record for this book has been requested.

ISBN 978 1 44730 111 0 paperback

Cover design by The Policy Press.
Front cover: image kindly supplied by istock.com
Printed and bound in Great Britain by MPG Book Group

FSC
www.fsc.org
MIX
From responsible sources
FSC® C018575

Contents

List of tables and figures

List of abbreviations

BHPS	British Household Panel Survey
BIS	Department for Business Innovation and Skills
CBT	Cognitive behavioural therapy
CIPD	Chartered Institute of Personnel and Development
CHD	Coronary heart disease
DB	Defined benefit pension
DC	Defined contribution pension
DCS	demand-control-support
DDA	Disability Discrimination Act
DH	Department of Health
DWP	Department for Work and Pensions
EHRC	Equality and Human Rights Commission
ELSA	English Longitudinal Study of Ageing
ERI	Effort-reward-imbalance
ESA	Employment Support Allowance
EU	European Union
FRS	Family Resources Survey
GDP	Gross domestic product
GHS	General Household Survey
GP	General practitioner
HRS	Health and Retirement Study
HRS	Health Retirement Survey (US)
HSE	Health and Safety Executive
IAPT	Improving Access to Psychological Therapies
IB	Incapacity Benefit
ILO	International Labour Organization
JSA	Jobseeker's Allowance
LFS	Labour Force Survey
LLSI	limiting long-standing illness
MRC	Medical Research Council
MSD	Musculoskeletal disorder
NAO	National Audit Office
NHS	National Health Service
NICE	National Institute for Health and Clinical Excellence
OECD	Organisation for Economic Co-operation and Development
ONS	Office for National Statistics
SCELI	Social Change and Economic Life Initiative

CMH	Centre for Mental Health (formerly Sainsbury Centre for Mental Health)
SDA	Severe Disablement Allowance
SEOW	South East Opportunities for Work
SWOT	Strengths, weaknesses, opportunities and threats
SPA	State pension ages
TAEN	The Age and Employment Network (formerly Third Age Employment Network)
VR	Vocational rehabilitation
WAI	Work Ability Index
WCA	Work Capability Assessment
WFI	Work-focused interview
WLD	Work-limiting disability
WHO	World Health Organization

Notes on contributors

Ben Baumberg is a lecturer in sociology and social policy at the University of Kent. The work is part of his thesis that links the changing nature of work, fitness for work and incapacity benefits receipt (see www.benbaumberg.com for updates). He also co-edits a collaborative blog on issues relating to social inequality (http://inequalitiesblog. wordpress.com)

Christina Beatty is a principal research fellow at the Centre for Regional Economic and Social Research (CRESR) at Sheffield Hallam University. She is a statistician by background and has published extensively on the social and economic geography of Britain, the growth of incapacity benefits over time and welfare reform. (www. shu.ac.uk/cresr/staff/c-beatty.html).

Rachel Black is a researcher in the Centre for Health Services Studies, University of Kent. Her research interests include suffering, emotion management and children's palliative care.

Michael Calnan is Professor of Medical Sociology, University of Kent. He has worked in health policy and health services research and training for over 20 years (m.w.calnan@ kent.ac.uk).

Steve Fothergill is a professor at CRESR and an economist by background. He has published extensively on urban and regional economic analysis and policy, shifts within the benefits system and the changing nature of labour markets across the UK over time (www.shu. ac.uk/cresr/staff/s-fothergill.html).

Julia Gibbs is a freelance researcher and consultant in Montreal, Canada. From 2002-05 she was a research fellow at the University of Edinburgh, investigating organisational change and health as well as resilience in economically disadvantaged communities. From 2005-08 she was a senior consultant with health and social policy consultancy Blake Stevenson, Edinburgh.

Annie Irvine is a research fellow in the Social Policy Research Unit at the University of York. Her research focuses on health, disability, employment and social security benefits. She has particular interest in mental health and employment, and in qualitative interview methods.

Susan Kenyon is a lecturer in qualitative research methods in the Centre for Health Services Studies, University of Kent. Her current research combines transport and social exclusion with a specific focus on the social policy implications of physical (im)mobility and (in)accessibility.

Tina Kowalski is a research associate and PhD candidate in the University of Edinburgh Business School. Her doctoral research is investigating the ways in which social support at work can affect employee wellbeing.

David Lain is a research fellow at the University of Brighton Business School (www.brighton.ac.uk/bbs/contact/details.php?uid=dl77).

Wendy Loretto is Professor of Organisational Behaviour at the University of Edinburgh Business School. She has published in the areas of organisational change, employee wellbeing and matters relating to wellbeing in later working life.

Tony Maltby is an honorary fellow at both the University of Sheffield and University of Leicester. He is currently working as a freelance social researcher and writer (t.maltby@sheffield.ac.uk).

Fehmidah Munir is a senior lecturer in psychology at Loughborough University. Her expertise is in managing common health problems at work, sickness absence and return to work.

Chris Phillipson is Professor of Applied Social Studies and Social Gerontology in the School of Sociology and Criminology at Keele University (www.keele.ac.uk/sociology/people/chrisphillipson).

Stephen Platt is Professor of Health Policy Research at the University of Edinburgh. His has a long-standing research interest in measuring and understanding mental wellbeing, and is involved in policy development and analysis relating to public mental health.

Joanne Ross is an independent occupational therapist with a professional portfolio including management consultancy, service development, clinical practice and applied research. She has a keen interest in mental health and work issues.

Sarah Vickerstaff is Professor of Work and Employment in the School of Social Policy, Sociology and Social Research at the University of Kent (www.kent.ac.uk/sspssr/staff/academic/vickerstaff.html).

David Wainwright is a health sociologist who studies the connections between illness and society. He is a senior lecturer in the Department for Health, University of Bath and convenes the Work, Health and Wellbeing Research Group at the university.

Elaine Wainwright is a social psychologist working as a researcher in the Department for Health, University of Bath. Her current research focuses on the negotiation of sickness certification for chronic pain conditions, and introduction of the new fit note.

Ross Wilkie is a Research Councils UK research fellow in epidemiology. He graduated as a physiotherapist and worked as a clinician, specialising in musculoskeletal conditions. In 2000, he joined Keele University and began his research career, which has focused on the impact of pain.

Acknowledgments

We would like to thank the Lifelong Health and Wellbeing Project for funding the Collaborative Development Network that brought together the authors who have contributed to this text (Award reference G0900038). Our thanks also to all who participated in and helped organise the network meetings. We are indebted to all the authors who agreed to contribute chapters. Finally, we also wish to note our appreciation for the editing support provided by Lynn Walford in producing the manuscript.

ONE

Work, health and wellbeing: an introduction

Sarah Vickerstaff, Chris Phillipson and Ross Wilkie

Policies to extend working life have become a central response to the development of ageing populations. Delaying retirement is viewed as a means of mitigating the effects of worsening demographic ratios whilst increasing financial resources for later life. Such policies are variously presented as an 'unavoidable obligation' (Reday-Mulvey, 2005, p 195), 'a fiscal and social imperative' (PwC, 2010) or simply part of an injunction that people should 'live longer and work longer' (OECD, 2006). According to *The Economist* (2009), retirement has been 'overdone'. Many European governments, including that in the UK, have moved to raise pension ages along with a range of other measures such as anti-age discrimination legislation. It is in this context that our ability to maintain the capacity of individuals with significant health conditions to remain in, or return to, work is increasingly under the spotlight. While the ageing population sharpens our concern for health and wellbeing at work, this volume is not limited to a consideration of older workers. The personal and social desirability of enabling people with health conditions to remain in work if they are able and want to do so is relevant across all working age groups. A number of reviews have highlighted the importance of 'good work' to lifelong health and wellbeing in work and into retirement (Waddell and Burton, 2006; Black, 2008; Royal College of Psychiatrists, 2008; Marmot, 2010). This is tempered, however, by the further finding of the Marmot review that 'more than three-quarters of the population do not have disability-free life expectancy as long as 68' (2010, p 17). In the UK, with the state pension age expected to rise to 68 by 2046, we can expect more and more people in work to be coping with a significant chronic health condition, in particular mental health issues and musculoskeletal disorders, which are the two big health concerns that compromise individuals' ability to work (Black, 2008).

It is clear that the impact of ill health on an individual's ability to remain in paid employment depends on complex interactions between biological, psychological, social and organisational factors. This edited collection seeks to explore these compound connections linking a variety of disciplines and professional groups. The volume's genesis arises from a collaborative, interdisciplinary network, established by the book's editors with funding from the Cross Research Council Life-Long Health and Wellbeing Initiative, which began meeting in April 2009. The aim of the network is to bring together a multidisciplinary group of academics and practitioners undertaking research in the area of managing health conditions at work, with particular reference to musculoskeletal disorders (MSDs) and mental health issues. It is from the network, with one exception, that the current collection is drawn. In this introduction, we provide an overview of the issues involved in managing health and wellbeing at work. The discussion is organised in four sections: the current context for interest in work and wellbeing issues; the developing policy context; existing research that seeks to understand the factors influencing the individual's ability or willingness to continue working with a health issue; and an introduction to the subsequent chapters.

The contemporary context

The ability to manage health conditions in order to continue in paid work has always been important for both the individuals whose health is compromised and the organisation that wants to retain them. In the days when a high proportion of the male workforce was engaged in physical labour, the emphasis was on health and safety at work and the prevention of accidents or injury in the workplace; with the move to a more service-based economy, attention has also focused on other concerns, such as stress, health promotion and wellbeing.

It is clear that there are many factors in the 21st century that make a focus on health and work of increasing importance for individuals, for employers and for governments. Three interrelated developments stand out as sharpening the need for better management of health at work: first, our increasing awareness and understanding of the relationship between work and health; second, trends in health patterns in the general population and in particular the persistently large number of people claiming Incapacity Benefit (IB); and third, the ageing population. We consider these in turn.

Health and work

The relationship between health and work is widely recognised as complex and multifaceted. In recent years, the traditional academic and practical splits between considerations of health and safety at work and wider considerations of wellbeing have begun to blur, recognising that work-related and lifestyle-related factors are often interconnected in producing healthy work, healthy workers and healthy citizens. The relationship between health and work is two-way: while good work is generally beneficial and unemployment tends to depress health, certain types of work can also pose a risk to wellbeing (Waddell and Burton, 2006; Marmot, 2010).

In this century, governments have become progressively convinced that work is in most cases good for people, and policy is increasingly directed to keeping people in work or getting them back into the labour market:

Evidence shows that work is generally good for your health and that often going back to work can actually aid a person's recovery. On the other hand, staying off work can lead to long-term absence and job loss with the risk of isolation, loss of confidence, mental health issues, de-skilling and social exclusion.[1]

Research indicates that early intervention for those with a health condition – either keeping them in work or getting them back to work quickly – is important in avoiding long-term incapacity for work (Campbell et al, 2007; Black, 2008; Royal College of Psychiatrists, 2008; Waddell et al, 2008; Bevan et al, 2009; NAO, 2009).

Self-rated health, which is a common way of trying to measure general health in the population at large, indicates that while a majority of people self-define as in very good or good health, there are significant variations between those in employment and those unemployed or inactive, and there are also significant differences across age groups and across occupations, as shown in Table 1.1 (Health, Work and Wellbeing Strategy Unit, 2010; see also Booker and Sacker, 2011). Research over many years has identified that there is a 'social gradient' in health, meaning that health inequalities mirror wider social inequalities (for example, Marmot, 2010). This is reinforced through labour market opportunities, where the poorest, least qualified sections of the population are most likely to experience low-quality paid employment, which is more insecure and potentially more prejudicial to health. The poorest are also, of course, more at risk of unemployment, which compounds the risk of ill health (Marmot, 2010, p 68).

The number of accidents at work in the UK continues to decline as larger proportions of the working population are engaged in service- and office-based sectors rather than manual and industrial occupations. Against this, the reporting of stress and mental health issues among the working population continues to rise (HSE, 2009b). The overall picture

Table 1.1: Self-reported general health, Britain, 2008

	Health in general (%)				
	Very good	Good	Fair	Bad	Very bad
Overall	38	41	16	4	1
Employment status					
Employed	48	42	9	1	0
Self-employed	45	43	11	1	0
ILO unemployed	33	45	18	4	1
Economically inactive	22	36	29	10	3
NS-SEC* (five-class version)					
Managerial and professional occupations	46	40	11	2	1
Intermediate occupations	38	42	16	4	1
Small employers and own account workers	34	43	17	4	1
Lower supervisory and technical occupations	31	43	17	6	2
Semi-routine occupations	31	39	21	7	1
Never worked and long-term unemployed	26	38	26	8	2
Not classified	54	38	7	1	0
Gender					
Male	39	41	15	4	1
Female	38	40	16	4	1
Age group					
16-24	53	40	7	1	0
25-34	52	40	6	1	0
35-44	49	39	10	2	1
45-54	37	44	14	4	1
55-64	32	42	20	6	1

Note: * National Statistics Socio-economic Classification.

Source: Health, Work and Well-being Strategy Unit (2010, p 23)

of ill health and injury among workers in the UK remains alarming: in 2008/09, 1.2 million people who had worked in the previous year reported suffering from an illness they felt was caused or made worse by their work. Some 29.3 million working days were lost due to workplace ill health or injury (HSE, 2009a).

While it is increasingly difficult to argue against the orthodoxy that 'work is good for you', it is clear that our understanding of the relationship between work and health needs to be nuanced, recognising that the relationship between a specific job in a particular organisation, the individual undertaking it or seeking to gain employment and their health is a dynamic one. Access to 'good work' is not equally available to all.

Health trends

There is considerable variance in health trends due to the different ways in which general health, illness and disability are operationalised (see Chapters Four and Five). One fact about which there is agreement is that we are living longer. There is evidence that while infectious diseases in countries like the UK do not wreak the dramatic public health consequences they did even a century ago, chronic disease and ill health are now major cause for concern in terms of individual wellbeing, and costs to both employers in sickness absence and the state with respect to healthcare and benefits. The major chronic illnesses in contemporary Britain are MSDs, which include arthritis and back pain; heart and circulatory conditions; respiratory conditions; and mild to moderate mental health disorders (see Tables 1.2 and 1.3). These long-term and often limiting conditions are more pronounced in the older population, but there are also some differences between women and men and across social classes (Royal College of Psychiatrists, 2008).

It has been recognised for some time in the UK that incapacity to work is numerically a more significant issue than unemployment, amounting to 7% of the total working-age population in 2010 (see Chapter Seven). The numbers of people claiming IB began to rise in

Table 1.2: Self-reported long-standing illness by age and gender, Britain, 2008

| | Rates per 1,000 population | | | | | | | |
| | Men | | | | Women | | | |
	16–44	45–64	65–74	75 and over	16–44	45–64	65–74	75 and over
Musculoskeletal								
Arthritis and rheumatism	11	64	114	118	15	97	193	236
Back problems	21	47	33	31	18	41	31	36
Other bone and joint problems	13	37	46	87	12	41	67	117
Heart and circulatory								
Heart attack	*	22	54	58	*	8	26	45
Stroke	1	6	24	33	*	6	16	27
Other heart complaints	4	50	110	117	5	23	59	111
Other blood vessel/embolic disorders	*	9	20	29	1	5	7	18
Respiratory								
Asthma	29	30	30	41	47	45	52	44
Bronchitis and emphysema	0	4	26	33	*	6	16	16
Hay fever	5	3	*	0	3	*	*	0
Other respiratory complaints	3	17	24	34	3	6	13	27

Source: ONS (2010, p 102)

Table 1.3: Prevalence of common mental disorders by gender, England, 2007

	Males (%)	Females (%)
Mixed anxiety and depressive disorders	6.9	11.0
Generalised anxiety disorder	3.4	5.3
Depressive episode	1.9	2.8
All phobias	0.8	2.0
Obsessive compulsive disorder	0.9	1.3
Panic disorder	1.0	1.2

Source: ONS (2010, p 104)

1980s and has plateaued. The two main health reasons for incapacity to work are mental ill health and MSDs, but the number of mental health cases seems to be on the rise (see Table 1.4). There is considerable debate as to why the numbers claiming IB have increased and then stabilised at a high level (see Chapters Five, Seven and Eight). What is agreed is that there are considerable difficulties in getting people back into work once they have been unemployed or incapacitated for a period of time, especially the older they are.

Table 1.4: Increasing trend of mental/behavioural ill health and disability as the medical basis of an incapacity claim, Britain

	Women		Men	
	2000	2007	2000	2007
Mental/behavioural	35.4	43.2	34.8	45.1
Musculoskeletal	22.4	18.4	19.1	14.5

Note: Data covers IB and Severe Disablement Allowance, claimants aged 16-59.
Source: Beatty et al (2009)

Ageing population

While the fact that we are living longer – and, for many, healthier – older lives should be a cause for celebration, it is increasingly tempered by concern. In particular, it is argued that an ageing population will unbalance the established intergenerational contract on which many welfare states are based – namely, that current prime-age workers pay for the pensions and healthcare of the retired. If this so-called 'dependency ratio' is fundamentally altered by increasing numbers of older people as a proportion of the total population, governments will face difficulties in how to finance education, pensions, healthcare and care services (see Table 1.5; and on current projections of the dependency ratio, see Pensions Commission 2004, ch 1; Dini, 2009, p 11).

Table 1.5: Dependency ratio: numbers of people of working age for every person of state pension age, UK

2008	2013	2018	2028	2033
3.23	3.19	3.11	3.07	2.78

Source: ONS (2009)

Across Europe, the ages at which people might normally expect to retire are rising for a number of reasons. In many countries, the age at which people can gain access to a state pension is being steadily raised, as are the normal retirement ages for public sector pension schemes (Independent Public Service Pension Commission, 2011). The value of many occupational and private pensions has been undermined in the economic turbulence of the second decade of the new century, meaning that people will have to work longer and continue contributing to a pension in order to approach the standard of living in retirement they had hoped for. Governments are generally encouraging people to work for longer by measures such as outlawing age discrimination, scrapping default retirement ages and making it financially attractive to defer take-up of state pensions. The employment rate of those over 65 has been increasing in the UK (see Table 1.6) and current trends suggest this will continue, although job losses in the current recession may temper this trend. As a result of these developments, there will be larger numbers of older workers in the labour force, with the corollary that more people are likely to be trying to combine continuing to work with a long-standing health condition.

Table 1.6: Employment rates (%) for men and women aged 50+, by age group, Britain

Age group	Men		Women	
	2004	2010	2004	2010
50-54	84	82.8	75	75.6
55-59	75	76.1	61	65.5
60-64	54	54.5	30	33.9
65-69	18	24.2	10	16.3
70+	4	4.9	2	2.7
Total 50+	45	44.5	31	33.1

Sources: 2004 (Loretto et al, 2005, p 9); 2010 LFS analysis by W. Loretto

The developing policy context

For much of the second half of the 20th century, the main pressure on governments and employers was in the health and safety arena, with an emphasis on the prevention of accidents and injury, and rehabilitation when they did occur. The focus was firmly on the workplace and the measurement and management of risks. With structural shifts in employment away from industry and towards services and other white-collar occupations and accompanying changes in employees' expectations, we have seen a slow but increasingly marked move towards a focus on health promotion and active management of ill health. The drivers for these changes have been various. For government, the rising tide of people claiming IB has concentrated the mind on how to keep people in work or get them back to employment. For employers, the costs of employee absence and insurance issues have begun to illustrate the business case for better management of health issues in the workplace (PwC, 2008; Bevan, 2010). In addition, as is often the case in other areas of human resource management, the example of large foreign owned multinationals, especially American-owned companies that have had employee health and wellbeing policies for some time, has a trickle-down effect on domestic companies (for a sense of the level of debate in the US, see Sibson Consulting, 2011). There is also arguably a change in social attitudes towards work, in part arising from the increasing numbers of women in the paid labour force. Work–life balance, time management, stress management and health promotion programmes have come to be expected elements of employment in large enterprises (PwC, 2008).

The costs of work-related illness and workplace injury are substantial, and, in addition, there are the working days lost through other forms of illness. It has been estimated that:

> The annual economic costs of sickness absence and worklessness associated with working age ill-health are estimated to be over £100 billion. This is greater than the current annual budget for the NHS and equivalent to the entire GDP of Portugal. (Black, 2008, p 10)

The costs are felt by individuals in lost earnings, by employers in lost productivity and illness-related costs such as sick pay and insurance, and by society in terms of medical treatment and benefits. Focusing on workplace accidents and work-related ill health, the Health and Safety Executive (HSE) has identified a number of different costs categories (see Figure 1.1, overleaf). The HSE estimation of costs to employers alone for 2005/06 was between £2.9 and £3.2 billion (HSE, 2008, p 5). This, coupled with government expenditure on health and welfare benefits for those unable to work, amounts to a strong argument for tackling work, health and wellbeing issues.

Two main strands of public policy have emerged in response to these pressures. The first is a move towards activation policies (Houston and Lindsay, 2010) or conditionality in welfare policy for those *out of work*. In this area, those unemployed or inactive for reasons of health or caring are increasingly expected to demonstrate a willingness to search for work, be rehabilitated or undertake training or work preparation as a condition of benefit receipt. The second strand is a more general public health focus on wellbeing aimed at those *in work*. Both aspects of policy are underpinned by the belief that work is beneficial in terms of health and social inclusion, as discussed earlier.

By the early years of the 21st century, the number of people on IB was seen as an increasingly intractable policy problem. Against a backdrop of the improving general health of the population and a reasonably buoyant labour market, the large number of people claiming such benefits was difficult to reconcile. The prevailing explanation in policy circles was in part that labour demand had changed, but more significantly that numbers of the unemployed were transferring to IB because of the 'the relative advantages of claiming incapacity benefits over the more demanding and less generous Jobseeker's Allowance' (NAO, 2010, p 14; see also Houston and Lindsay, 2010). The New Labour government became committed to reducing the numbers of people claiming IB. In 2003, a new Pathways to Work programme was piloted in seven areas before being rolled out nationally by 2008 (Lindsay and Dutton, 2010). The main features of the Pathways to Work programme was a more individualised or person-centred approach, with the claimant being required to attend work-focused interviews, and having access to work preparation and possible voluntary involvement in a condition management programme (Lindsay and Dutton, 2010).

In 2005, two government departments, the Department of Health (DH) and the DWP, came together with the Health and Safety Executive (HSE) to produce the joint report *Health, work and well-being – caring for our future*, which made a commitment to:

> improve the health of the working age population and minimise the risk of employees becoming ill in the first place; improve employee retention by supporting them during periods of transition; and build a world

Figure 1.1: Cost categories

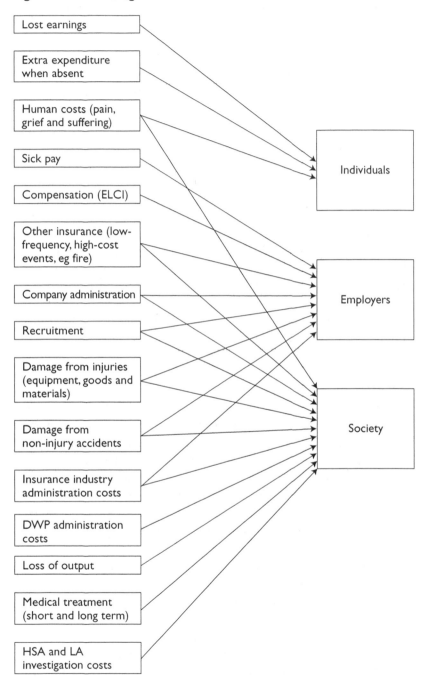

Note: ELCI = Employers Liability Compulsory Insurance; LA= Local Authorities
Source: Health and Safety Executive (2004)

which rehabilitates rather than rejects people when they experience illness or disability. In this way we can support individuals to fulfil their potential in contributing to society. We can enable employers and the economy as a whole to gain from the huge potential that our people have to offer, and we can also deliver on our responsibility as a society, to ensure equal rights and opportunity for all. (DWP, DH and HSE, 2005, p 3)

Carol Black was appointed as the National Director for Health and Work and was commissioned to undertake a review of the health of the working-age population (Black, 2008). A number of policy developments resulted from the government's response to the Black Report (DWP and DH, 2008):

- the switch from April 2010 to the fit note, which replaced the old sick note through which GPs would sign people off work;
- a review of the health and wellbeing of the NHS workforce (Boorman, 2009);
- a national strategy for mental health and employment (DWP, 2009);
- the development of a Business health check tool;[2]
- occupational health advice lines for small and medium-sized enterprises; and
- the development of a pilot Fit for Work Service.

The move to a fit note system had been developing for some time, along with changes to in access to disability benefits. In 2006, the DWP commissioned the Health, Work and Wellbeing Directorate to review the personal capability assessment (PCA), the tool used to assess entitlement to IB, the focus being on developing a more 'positive assessment, focusing on capability and on health-related interventions which could contribute to overcoming the barriers preventing people with disabilities from engaging in work' (DWP, 2006). Following the 2007 Welfare Reform Act, a work capability assessment (WCA) was introduced from October 2008. IB was subsequently replaced by the Employment Support Allowance (ESA). The WCA divides new claimants into three groups: those able to work, those who could work in the future with some support (the work-related activity group) and those who cannot work (the support group). Early indications suggest that the WCA is a stiffer test than the old PCA and more claimants are being defined as capable of work either straight away or with support. The new fit note is designed to encourage health professionals to focus on what the patient can do rather than assuming that illness necessarily precludes work. As a DWP information leaflet for health professionals comments:

> The new Statement of Fitness for Work has been designed to help you to provide more information on the functional effects of your patient's condition and to allow you to suggest options that would facilitate a return to work. You do not need specialist occupational health expertise or a detailed understanding of your patient's job to complete the form. The advice you give is on the functional effects of the condition within the limits of your knowledge and expertise. This advice will help your patient's employer to make a more active contribution to your patient's recovery.[3]

Ten Fit for Work Service pilot areas were commissioned to trial partnership approaches to helping people with health issues to stay in work or get back into work more quickly, providing case management support covering healthcare, employment advice, employer liaison, learning and skills advice and wider social support such as debt or housing advice as appropriate in each case. The pilots often built on existing services and ran with public pump priming funds until March 2011.[4]

In 2006, the NHS began with two demonstration sites for an Improving Access to Psychological Therapies (IAPT) programme for people of working age suffering from depression and anxiety disorders. In 2007, 11 IAPT Pathfinder projects were commissioned and the programme was rolled out nationally from.[5] Cognitive and behavioural therapy (CBT) is the preferred method of therapy under the IAPT schemes and since the initiative began there has been a boost in the numbers of people trained to offer CBT interventions.

From these various policy developments, we can see that there has been movement on several fronts to make it more difficult for people to be simply signed off as sick or incapable of work. Efforts have been made to restructure health professional and employer roles in managing ill health and individuals face stiffer conditionality tests in order to receive benefits. IAPT, Pathways to Work and pilot Fit for Work Services have led to a generally more interventionist approach and growing body of knowledge as to what works in getting people back into work, although the National Audit Office value for money audit of the Pathways programme concluded that 'Pathways is not having the level of impact on the employment of claimants of incapacity benefits suggested by pilot results' (NAO, 2010, p 12).

The NAO review indicated that a slight drop in the numbers of people coming on to ESA was down to the new WCA rather than access to Pathways provisions (NAO, 2010). An independent review of the WCA has argued that its operation is sometimes 'impersonal and mechanistic' and that some conditions such as mental health issues may be more difficult to assess than others (Harrington, 2010).

In response to the Harrington review of WCA, the coalition government reiterated the commitment to moving people off ESA:

> From April 2011 we will put 1.6 million people, all of those on incapacity benefits who are not close to retirement, through an independent medical assessment. Those found fit for work or with the potential to return to work will be given specialist support to help them do so, through Jobcentre Plus and through our new Work Programme. Those who are deemed unable to work will continue to receive full support. (DWP, 2010a, p 5)

The Work Programme is the coalition government's flagship welfare-to-work plan, which will replace New Labour's employment programmes under the New Deals banner. The policy continues the trend toward conditionality in benefits and the design and delivery of employment support programmes will be in the hands of public, private and voluntary agencies (DWP, 2010b). It was also announced in February 2011 that there would be an independent review of how sickness absence systems could be changed to help people stay in work, to be chaired by David Frost, Director General of the British Chambers of Commerce, and Dame Carol Black, National Director for Health and Work.

In the first decade of the 21st century, public policy has increasingly focused on how to change the behaviour of individuals, employers and health professionals in the management of ill health. We turn now to a consideration of the understanding of illness, which underpins these developments.

The 'illness experience': understanding the factors that encourage or inhibit continuing to work

Central to all attempts to manage health and work is our understanding of the 'illness experience' and the factors likely to encourage or inhibit continuing to work. Running alongside the policy developments detailed in the previous section, there has been growing research on, and support for, a biopsychosocial model of the illness experience as the most effective basis for rehabilitation (see, for example, Waddell and Burton, 2004; Seymour and Grove, 2005; Campbell et al, 2007). Waddell and Burton (2004, p 19) define a biopsychosocial approach:

> Put simply, this is an individual-centred model that considers the person, their health problem, *and* their social context:
>
> > *Biological* refers to the physical or mental health condition. (By definition, everyone receiving a disability or incapacity benefit has been diagnosed by a medical practitioner as having a physical or mental disease or disablement. However, this does *not* imply that the biopsychosocial model is simply an extended medical model).
> >
> > *Psychological* recognises that personal/psychological factors also influence functioning and the individual must take some measure of personal responsibility for his or her behaviour. (It does *not* imply that the person is 'mad' or that 'it is in their head').
> >
> > *Social* recognises the importance of the social context, pressures and constraints on behaviour and functioning. (Social interactions are two-way between the individual and his or her environment, but some of these factors are environmental and must be addressed by society).
> >
> > The biopsychosocial model is particularly relevant to common health problems, where rehabilitation must address *all* of the biological, personal/psychological, and social dimensions. (Emphasis in original.)

Translating this model into the employment context means that we need to explain the interaction of organisational, individual and social factors in the management of wellbeing in the workplace, which includes the connections between:

- medical diagnosis and symptoms;
- organisational policies and processes relating to health, illness and wellbeing;
- working conditions;

- life events;
- individual characteristics;
- beliefs around health and work, embedded in the social environment; and
- social support inside and outside the workplace.

Reviews of the success of different types of intervention to keep people in work or get them to return to employment have argued for multidisciplinary programmes that take a biopsychosocial approach:

> Biopsychosocial support was defined as including elements which aim to increase activity level and restore function (biological), change behaviour, shift perceptions, attitudes and beliefs in personal and work life (psychological), and support with involvement of employer where possible (social). (Campbell et al, 2007, p 51)

The precise combination of interventions and the specific professional input needed obviously depends on the individual case, the specific health issue and its severity (Waddell et al, 2008). It is clear from the literature that keeping people with health issues in work requires complex and often multilayered interventions that require the involvement of different agencies. A comprehensive literature review of what works in vocational rehabilitation concluded:

> Many stakeholders have an interest in work and health: workers, employers, trade unions, insurers, health professionals, policy makers and government. For most short-term sickness absence, the key players in the return to work process are the worker/patient, GP and employer. For longer-term sickness absence, vocational rehabilitation may involve a more extensive list of players: which may include any combination of the worker/patient, GP and primary care team, employer, occupational health, rehabilitation team, insurer, case manager, and DWP Personal Adviser. Different stakeholders have different perspectives, agendas and budgets, which are not always aligned. Vocational rehabilitation interventions will only be successful if the various players work together and not at cross-purposes. And the development of vocational rehabilitation policy depends on keeping all stakeholders onside. (Waddell et al, 2008, p 40)

It is clear from this that while there is now broad agreement about the approaches needed to manage work, health and wellbeing more effectively, we are still at a relatively early stage in mobilising the different stakeholders to play their part. This volume seeks to contribute to this process by identifying some of the key theoretical and practical hurdles yet to be negotiated.

Contributions in this volume

In the chapters that follow, a range of research is presented that tackles various aspects of work, health and wellbeing. The contributors come from a number of different academic disciplines and are all researchers and/or practitioners in the field. Chapters Two (Ross Wilkie) and Three (Annie Irvine) examine the health issues that dominate the statistics for working days lost and reasons for incapacity to work: musculoskeletal disorders and common mental health problems. Both chapters outline the scale and the nature of the problems in these areas of ill health and review what helps in managing these conditions. Chapter Four by David Lain focuses on the influence of health and wealth on employment past 65, comparing the US and England. This raises questions of how to assess the impact of health on employment and the selection of suitable health measures. The theme of measurement is taken up again in Chapter Five when Ben Baumberg considers various definitions of disability and argues that in relation to ability to work it may be more revealing to focus and measure *work-limiting* disability rather than disability per se. The centrality of vocational rehabilitation (VR) services to improving the management of health at work is highlighted in Chapter Six, where Joanne Ross provides an overview of the current state of VR services in the UK, looking both at contemporary approaches to VR, including traditional condition-focused and newer occupation-focused perspectives, and the contexts in which services are delivered.

As evidenced earlier, the persistently high number of people on IB has been a major driver for public policy development in the health, work and wellbeing arena and Chapters Seven and Eight look specifically at IB recipients. In Chapter Seven, Christina Beatty and Steve Fothergill argue that understanding just who makes up the stock of incapacity claimants is very significant in targeting effective policy, and they also pose the question of the extent to which the profile of claimants has stayed the same or changed. This is important, because although we know that the numbers on IB have remained high, we have a less clear picture of the new cohorts coming on to benefits. In Chapter Eight,

David Wainwright and colleagues report on a qualitative study that explores the effectiveness of current interventions to support the return to work for long-term IB recipients. This contribution reminds us of the value of looking at the user experience of interventions.

In Chapter Nine, David Wainwright and Michael Calnan critique the notion of work stress and chart the rise of the new wellbeing at work agenda, arguing for a definition of wellbeing that gives some agency back to the employee. In Chapter Ten, Tony Maltby provides an exploration of the influential Finnish Work Ability model and considers its potential as an approach in the UK.

The following three chapters move into the workplace to look at a number of different dimensions of work experience. In Chapter Eleven, Fehmidah Munir looks at how employees can seek to self-manage their own health conditions and be facilitated in doing so by the organisation they work for. Next, in Chapter Twelve, Julia Gibbs and colleagues provide a case study investigating the impact of organisational change in the NHS on employees' health and wellbeing. As organisational change is now considered to be virtually continuous, this chapter argues that managing change successfully is an important backdrop to promoting employee health and wellbeing. Finally, in Chapter Thirteen, Chris Phillipson returns to the issue of an ageing workforce and the extending working life agenda. Focusing on the known fact that older workers are less likely to receive training and professional development than younger colleagues, the chapter makes the link between education and training and health and wellbeing in the workplace.

In the Conclusion, the editors draw the volume together by outlining the main research agendas identified in the various chapters. Five areas are highlighted: developing work across different types of organisations; improving the work environment; developing effective interventions; developing a user perspective; and securing effective multidisciplinary/multi-centre studies. The chapter ends with a summary of some of the main challenges for delivering effecting health and well-being policies in the workplace.

Notes

[1] Department for Work and Pensions fit note website (www.dwp.gov.uk/fitnote).

[2] www.businesslink.gov.uk/bdotg/action/detail?itemId=1084516235&type=PIP&furlname=wwt&furlparam=wwt

[3] www.dwp.gov.uk/docs/fitnote-gp-guide.pdf

[4] See www.dwp.gov.uk/health-work-and-well-being/our-work/fit-for-work-services

[5] See the NHS IAPT website, www.iapt.nhs.uk/iapt

Further reading

Bevan, S., Quadrello, T., McGee, R., Mahdon, M., Vavrosky, A. and Barham, L. (2009) *Fit for work? Musculoskeletal disorders in the European workforce*, London: The Work Foundation.

Black, C. (2008) *Working for a healthier tomorrow*, London: The Stationery Office.

Marmot, M., Allen, J., Goldblatt, P., Boyce, T., McNeish, D., Grady, M. and Geddes, I. (2010) *Fair society, healthy lives: The Marmot review, strategic review of health inequalities in England post-2010*, London: Department of Health.

Royal College of Psychiatrists (2008) *Mental health at work*, London: Royal College of Psychiatrists.

Waddell, G. and Burton, A.K. (2006) *Is work good for your health and well-being?*, London: The Stationery Office.

References

Beatty, C., Fothergill, S., Houston, D., Powell, R. and Sissons, P. (2009) 'Women on incapacity benefits: a statistical overview', Unpublished paper.

Bevan, S. (2010) *The business case for employee health and wellbeing*, London: The Work Foundation.

Bevan, S., Quadrello, T., McGee, R., Mahdon, M., Vavrosky, A. and Barham, L. (2009) *Fit for work? Musculoskeletal disorders in the European workforce*, London: The Work Foundation.

Black, C. (2008) *Working for a healthier tomorrow*, London: The Stationery Office.

Booker, C.L. and Sacker, A. (2011) *Health over the life course: associations between age, employment status and well-being*, Early Findings from the First Wave of the UK'S Household Longitudinal Study. Colchester: Institute for Social and Economic Research, University of Essex.

Boorman, S. (2009) *NHS health and wellbeing*, London: Department of Health.

Campbell, J., Wright, C., Moseley, A., Chilvers, R., Richards, S. and Stabb, L. (2007) *Avoiding long-term incapacity for work: Developing an early intervention in primary care*, Exeter: Peninsula Medical School.

DWP (2006) 'Transformation of the personal capability assessment', http://www.dwp.gov.uk/docs/tpca.pdf

DWP (2009) *Realising the ambition: Better employment support for people with mental health conditions*, Cm 7742, London: The Stationery Office.

DWP (2010a) *Government's response to Professor Malcolm Harrington's independent review of the work capability assessment*, Cm 7977, London: The Stationery Office.

DWP (2010b) *Universal credit: Welfare that works*, Cm 7957, London: The Stationery Office.

DWP and DH (2008) *Improving health and work: Changing lives. The government's response to Dame Carol Black's review of the health of Britain's working-age population*, Cm 7492, London: The Stationery Office.

DWP, DH and HSE (2005) *Health, work and well-being – caring for our future*, London: The Stationery Office.

Dini, E. (2009) 'Older workers in the UK: variations in economic activity status by socio-demographic characteristics, household and caring commitments', *Population Trends*, vol 137, pp 11-24.

Harrington, M. (2010) *An independent review of the work capability assessment*, London: The Stationery Office.

HSE (Health and Safety Executive) (2004) 'Interim update of the "Costs to Britain of workplace accidents and work-related ill health"', www.hse.gov.uk/economics/costs.pdf

HSE (2008) 'The costs to employers in Britain of workplace injuries and work-related ill-health in 2005/06' Discussion Paper Series, No. 002, available at www.hse.gov.uk/economics/research/injuryill0506.pdf

HSE (2009a) *Health and Safety Statistics 2008/09*, Sudbury: HSE Books, available at www.hse.gov.uk/statistics/overall/hssh0809.pdf

HSE (2009b) 'Historical picture. Workplace injury and ill health trends following the introduction of the Health and Safety at Work Act 1974', http://www.hse.gov.uk/statistics/history/index.htm

Health, Work and Well-being Strategy Unit (2010) 'Health, work and well-being: Baseline indicators report', www.dwp.gov.uk/docs/hwwb-baseline-indicators.pdf

Houston, D. and Lindsay, C. (2010) 'Fit for work? Health, employability and challenges for the UK welfare reform agenda', *Policy Studies*, vol 31, no 2, pp 133-42.

Independent Public Service Pension Commission (2011) *Final report*, London: The Stationery Office.

Lindsay, C. and Dutton, M. (2010) 'Employability through health? Partnership-based governance and the delivery of Pathways to Work condition management services', *Policy Studies*, vol 31, no 2, pp 245-64.

Loretto W, Vickerstaff S, and White P (2005) *Older workers and Options for Flexible Work*. Manchester: Equal Opportunities Commission.

Marmot, M., Allen, J., Goldblatt, P., Boyce, T., McNeish, D., Grady, M. and Geddes, I. (2010) *Fair society, healthy lives: The Marmot review, strategic review of health inequalities in England post-2010,* London: Department of Health.

NAO (National Audit Office) (2009) *Services for people with rheumatoid arthritis,* London: The Stationery Office.

NAO (2010) *Support to incapacity benefits claimants through Pathways to Work,* London: The Stationery Office.

ONS (Office for National Statistics) (2009) 'National population projections 2008-based' *Statistical bulletin,* www.statistics.gov.uk/pdfdir/pproj1009.pdf.

ONS (2010) 'Social trends 40', www.statistics.gov.uk/downloads/theme_social/Social-Trends40/ST40_2010_FINAL.pdf.

OECD (Organisation for Economic Co-operation and Development) (2006) *Live longer, work longer,* Paris: OECD.

Pensions Commission (2004) *Pensions: Challenges and choices: The first report of the Pensions Commission,* London: The Stationery Office.

PwC (PricewaterhouseCoopers) (2008) *Building the case for wellness,* www.workingforhealth.gov.uk/documents/dwp-wellness-report-public.pdf.

PwC (2010) *Working longer, living better: A fiscal and social imperative,* http://psrc.pwc.com/html/gbclient/content/premium/communities/psrc/publications/working_longer_living_better.html

Reday-Mulvey, G. (2005) *Working beyond 60,* Basingstoke: Palgrave Macmillan.

Royal College of Psychiatrists (2008) *Mental health at work,* London: Royal College of Psychiatrists.

Seymour, L. and Grove, B. (2005) *Workplace interventions for people with common mental health problems: Evidence, review and recommendations,* London: British Occupational Health Research Foundation.

Sibson Consulting (2011) 'Results from Sibson's Healthy Enterprise Study', www.sibson.com/publications/surveysandstudies/HEall.pdf

The Economist (2009) 'Special report on ageing populations', 27 June, p 9.

Waddell, G. and Burton, A.K. (2004) *Concepts of rehabilitation for the management of common health problems,* London: The Stationery Office.

Waddell, G. and Burton, A.K. (2006) *Is work good for your health and well-being?,* London: The Stationery Office.

Waddell, G., Burton, A.K. and Kendall, N.A.S. (2008) *Vocational rehabilitation: What works, for whom, and when?,* London: The Stationery Office.

TWO

Musculoskeletal disorders: challenges and opportunities

Ross Wilkie

The impact of musculoskeletal disorders on work is demanding more attention from stakeholders, including clinicians and policymakers. Musculoskeletal disorders are the most frequently cited reason for absence from work (Black, 2008). Dame Carol Black's report *Working for a healthier tomorrow* (Black, 2008) and the subsequent government response *Improving health and work: Changing lives* (DWP and DH, 2008) highlight the need for new approaches and attitudes to assess and reduce the burden. National policies directed at extending working life further increase this need. The incidence and prevalence of many musculoskeletal disorders increase with age. Extensions to working life will result in greater numbers of older adults in the workplace with musculoskeletal disorders and associated disability. Significantly, new approaches impose the view that work loss does not need to be a consequence of a musculoskeletal disorder or disability. This presents an achievable challenge to everyone and underlines the importance of a biopsychosocial and interdisciplinary approach involving interaction between those with a musculoskeletal condition, employers, clinicians and policymakers.

This chapter provides an overview of the link between musculoskeletal disorders and work. It is not exhaustive, but provides examples of the evolving approach to musculoskeletal disorders and work and outlines the challenges to, and opportunities for, improving work participation. In the first instance, it reinforces the size of the burden of musculoskeletal disorders, and summarises the current health and employer approaches to improving work participation. Importantly, the discussion moves on to outline future research questions to maintain the current momentum and interest in reducing the burden of musculoskeletal disorders on work.

The burden of musculoskeletal conditions on work

Much attention is given to stress and mental health problems because they account for the majority of time absent from work. However, musculoskeletal disorders account for a rather higher number of episodes of absence from work. In the United Kingdom in 2007, 9.5 million working days were lost, with the cost estimated at £7.4 billion (Black, 2008). The level of morbidity is perhaps not reflected in the priority given to musculoskeletal disorders for their effective prevention and treatment by clinicians and policymakers, and for research to advance understanding (Woolf, 2000). Why are they ignored or underestimated? Because it is a common belief first, that we have to learn to live with musculoskeletal pain and disability as part of the ageing process and second, that nothing can be done to change the condition or its impact, which prevents planning and access to effective management. Both of these beliefs are incorrect. Musculoskeletal disorders are not caused by ageing, but as we get older, some predisposing factors (for example, increasing weight, less physical activity) increase and the risk of developing a condition heightens, along with the risk of that condition progressing. Many causes of musculoskeletal disorders may be prevented and there is a growing list of potential interventions that can reduce the symptoms and manage the disorder itself. The frequency of musculoskeletal disorders demand a response for better care and management; musculoskeletal disorders are:

- the most common cause of severe long-term pain (Woolf and Pfelger, 2003);
- the dominant cause of physical limitation in older people (Woolf and Pfelger, 2003);
- associated with an increased risk of mental health problems (Woolf and Pfelger, 2003);
- a significant burden on healthcare systems (WHO, 2003).

Musculoskeletal disorders are not homogenous and vary depending on cause and anatomical location. All have a muscle, joint, bone or nerve element and some – those that arise from an autoimmune response (for example, rheumatoid arthritis) – have a systemic component where many other tissues and organs can be affected. It is worth discussing the autoimmune disorders first of all. Rheumatoid arthritis is the most common autoimmune disorder and at present there are around 690,000 people with the condition in the United Kingdom, with 12,000 new diagnoses every year (Symmons et al, 2002; NAO, 2009).

While for a minority of people the disease is less severe and remains well controlled, others experience disabling pain, stiffness and reduced joint function, which have a huge impact on their work, their quality of life and that of their families (National Rheumatoid Arthritis Society, 2003;Young et al, 2005). Later in this chapter, the numerous co-morbid and psychosocial factors that combine with musculoskeletal disorders to affect work will be summarised, but it is important to highlight to policymakers the importance of medicines to manage autoimmune disorders and maintain work participation. Disease-modifying drugs are vastly improving the quality of life for patients with these conditions; by directly modifying the pathophysiology of the disorder, the signs and symptoms are reduced, with less pain and swelling. There are a number of studies (for example, Bejarano et al, 2008; Anis et al, 2009) that demonstrate their role in improving work outcomes, and rheumatologists are becoming increasingly aware that positive work outcomes are useful when justifying current, and requesting increased, resources for drugs to manage patients with autoimmune disorders. It is hoped that the National Institute for Health and Clinical Excellence will continue to take note of the wider societal costs when undertaking healthcare economic modelling to determine the cost-effectiveness of clinically effective, but expensive, new drugs.

Although the impact on the individual is often much greater, the cumulative burden of non-inflammatory arthropathies and disorders such as back pain, osteoarthritis and limb pain as a whole results in a much greater economic and human cost to society than autoimmune disease. Low back pain affects over one third of adults at any one time, and each year approximately 3.5 million people in the UK develop back pain (Maniadakis and Gray, 2000). It is the most common reason for middle-aged people to visit their general practitioner, with approximately 6-9% of adults consulting for this condition each year (Dunn and Croft, 2005). Although many back pain patients stop consulting their GP within three months, 60–80% of people still report pain or disability a year later, and up to 40% of those who have taken time off work will have future episodes of work absence (Croft et al, 1998; Hestbaek et al, 2003). Osteoarthritis and joint pain is the most common musculoskeletal condition in middle-aged to older adults (WHO, 2003). In North Staffordshire, 36% of adults aged 50 to 59 reported having knee pain for one day or more in the previous 12 months, one quarter reported hip pain and just under one quarter reported hand pain (Thomas et al, 2004). Notably, only around a third of these will seek healthcare (Jinks et al, 2004). As stated previously, people's perception of their condition make them reluctant to seek help, along with their experiences of primary care and secondary care, sustaining the pessimism about availability and effectiveness of treatments (Sanders et al, 2004). It would appear that in addition to the new approach that work need not be a consequence of musculoskeletal conditions, we should also highlight the need for new attitudes to the management of musculoskeletal disorders and that there are ways to reduce their impact and improve work participation and general function.

These disorders threaten the success of policies to extend working life because their incidence and prevalence increase with age; as working lives extend, there will be many more employees with musculoskeletal problems in years to come. The factors and mechanisms linked to work problems for older adults with musculoskeletal disorders are numerous:

- Pain is the key characteristic of musculoskeletal disorders and is strongly linked to loss of physical function in addition to age-associated functional decline (Jinks et al, 2007).
- Musculoskeletal pain is also linked to mental health problems (Williamson and Schulz, 1992). In particular, many patients with musculoskeletal pain also suffer from depression (Druss et al, 2000), which is a key factor for developing chronic disabling pain (Linton and Andersson, 2000). This combination is associated with increased absence from work (Currie and Wang, 2004) and interventions, which reduce depression severity in those with chronic pain, increase return to work (Sullivan et al, 2008).
- Co-morbidity increases with age and is even more common in those with musculoskeletal pain (WHO, 2003). Recent findings suggest that management strategies for musculoskeletal pain disorders should include consideration of these co-morbidities (Lee and Tracey, 2010).
- Psychological factors such as negative illness beliefs impact on perceptions of pain and work capacity (Main et al, 2007).
- Occupational factors can help to keep older adults with musculoskeletal pain in work (for example, through workplace accommodation) or increase absence and reduce productivity (for example, through high work demands and stress) (Franche et al, 2005).
- Socioeconomic factors are linked incidence and progression of pain and to health behaviour, which will have a bearing on working patterns in older adults (Marmot et al, 2010).

Improving work capability in older adults with musculoskeletal pain requires a multifactorial approach that addresses physical, psychological, social and occupational factors and focuses on managing the condition and associated co-morbidities rather than treating or 'curing' the condition (Waddell, 2006). This is important, as most people with musculoskeletal disorders have the potential to continue to work despite the persistence of symptoms.

Managing musculoskeletal disorders and work

The approach to managing musculoskeletal conditions and work is evolving. A coherent and effective response to the worker's need for support in continuing to work or returning to work is necessary. A greater emphasis on a 'joined-up' approach to the sick worker's problems involving the worker, the multidisciplinary team (for example, the GP, physiotherapist, occupational therapist, psychologist, occupational health professional, and/or employer adviser) and the employer is required.

The role of health professionals

The first point of contact in the United Kingdom for most people seeking help for a musculoskeletal problem is the National Health Service (NHS) and primary care, but is the current system flexible enough to respond to their needs and facilitate continued participation in work? Greater emphasis has been placed on early intervention, which is essential if a short-term problem is not to be translated into long-term sickness absence. Early diagnosis and treatment are key, but even at the early stage, the approach needs to incorporate a view of the problem wider than the purely medical by, for example, incorporating the evidence that patients' perceptions and emotional state are powerful predictors of whether they will return to work or not (Shaw et al, 2007). This highlights the current problem of access to key services (such as physiotherapy), which is restricted by resources and staff shortages. The aspiration to provide an early intervention service for dealing with musculoskeletal disorders will provide a challenge to the NHS, which has an ongoing struggle to meet existing demand. Waiting times for patients with musculoskeletal disorders have been historically high, although over the past 15 years these have been considerably reduced, providing quicker access to treatment for those in work. Increased involvement of allied health professionals to enhance patient care and reduce the pressure on general practitioners should be welcomed and encouraged, where, for example, a physiotherapist could make an assessment and refer on to colleagues appropriately (Campbell et al, 2008). The initial findings from a study of self-referral to physiotherapy in Scotland are encouraging (Holdsworth et al, 2007). Those who self-referred were likely to have a musculoskeletal condition and be in paid employment. Self-referral was found to be appropriate and resulted in a reduction in the number of contacts with general practitioners and other health professionals; the average cost benefit to NHS Scotland was approximately £2 million per year (Holdsworth et al, 2007). The increased savings for employers were not estimated, but the efficacy for early physiotherapy intervention is encouraged in the Boorman review to enhance health and wellbeing of NHS workers (Boorman, 2009).

Sickness certification has previously been a barrier to maintaining work participation; the 'sick note' or MED3 form only required the reason for absence to be given. The new 'fit note' directs a focus from absence to attendance and from incapacity to ability, and represents a marked improvement, but places new demands on general practitioners. They need to consider working-age patients as workers as much as people with an illness, explore their occupational practices (tasks involved and expectations for completion) and consider their environment (for example, employers' attitudes and capacity for supporting sick or disabled workers), to provide advice and for appropriate completion of the new fit note. This highlights a need for training and support, particularly for general practitioners who manage most working-age adults with musculoskeletal conditions. Such training will need to increase awareness of the solutions and support mechanisms that will assist employees to sustain participation in work or return to work and manage potential conflicts that this new approach may cause during consultation (Cooper, 2010). Identifying work-related problems may be as simple as directly asking about work absence and performance, but may require more systematic approaches, using existing tools that allow patients or workers to report work performance, ability and barriers. The Work Limitation Questionnaire (Lerner et al, 2001), Work Instability Scale (Gilworth et al, 2003) and the Work Experience Survey-Rheumatic Conditions (WES-RC) (Allaire and Keysor, 2009) have been developed to aid clinicians to identify work limitation and the barriers that may impede resolution. These could potentially become part of routine information gathering before, during or after the consultation.

Ideally, there should be a readily accessible and responsive occupational health service to which a general practitioner may refer the patient and this is one part of the developing relationship between clinicians and employers. Occupational health services are currently more likely to be found in association with larger employers. Support for smaller and medium-sized employers (which in 2007 employed 13.7 million people in the United Kingdom) is welcome to facilitate provision of more effective and supportive occupational health services, but at present this is the NHS. Vocational rehabilitation may have a greater role in the light of evidence of its benefits for employees and employers. There are various interventions that may help to keep people in work or aid return to work (Waddell et al, 2008). Many with the best evidence are primarily employer–based, and often involve interaction with the healthcare system, again highlighting the need for a strong link.

The Fit for Work pilots are currently ongoing and plan to evaluate a number of models aimed at helping people who develop a musculoskeletal disorder or other health condition to stay in or return to work. The aim of each model is to reduce absenteeism and ten centres have been chosen, each with a different approach, that build on existing attempts to manage work absence and focus on the health condition and the response of the health system.[1] For example, in North Staffordshire the pilot study tests the success of the expansion of an existing condition management programme to help unemployed people with musculoskeletal problems to return to work; this programme focuses on health issues that are important to individuals and promotes self-efficacy, capacity, confidence and empowerment to facilitate sustained participation in or return to work. It involves an interdisciplinary approach where health professionals link with Jobcentre Plus, employment specialists and training/educational centres. Another example is in Leicestershire, where one of the aims is to optimise GP referrals for employed people who are on, or at risk of, long-term sickness absence and unemployed people with health problems to case-managed fit-for-work schemes, so that this becomes routine practice. In addition, the Leicestershire Fit for Work Service also accepts referrals from practice therapists. Those referred are supported (one to one) by a case manager (with a vocational rehabilitation background) and occupational health nurses, GP and occupational health medicine specialists as required. There is access to a range of interventions including musculoskeletal care, talking therapies, career counselling, and debt and legal advice. There is promise that these interventions will prove useful, but careful evaluation of outcomes is required prior to more widespread implementation. Importantly, each model again highlights the importance of employer engagement.

The role of the employer

This evolving work agenda means a greater role for employers. The success of the new approach partly rests on the ability of clinicians to match 'accommodations', which could be in the form of a phased return, flexible hours, amended duties or workplace adaptation to the patient or worker's needs. Appropriate workplace accommodations are effective for enabling return to work, preventing work loss and disability, reducing related costs and the likelihood of subsequent work absence (Franche et al, 2005). But this is very much dependent on the willingness and the ability of employers to offer such accommodations. In the case of both short-term and long-term musculoskeletal disorders, opportunities to maintain work participation and productivity will be lost unless managers and employers can be more flexible and accommodating in their approach to the employee's condition. So the success of the new approach is perhaps more dependent on employers than on clinicians. Indeed, most people with a short-term work disability should be able to return to work without the involvement of any specialised services such as occupational health or vocational rehabilitation services. The most important interaction is between the employee and employer, and only when this is problematic should a return-to-work coordinator be needed (Pransky et al, 2004).

Occupational barriers and policies may restrict the ability of workers with musculoskeletal conditions to stay in work. The role of line managers, return-to-work coordinators and human resource departments, and their interaction with healthcare professions, will become increasingly important and crucial to the success of this initiative. Line managers need to consider the symptoms and functional limitations of such workers to optimise their performance. However, reducing absenteeism, and managing return to work and presenteeism, may depend more on competencies in ergonomic job accommodation, communication and conflict resolution than on direct management of the medical condition (Shaw et al, 2009). At an organisational level, again as is the case for the ability to provide in-house healthcare, large employers may be better placed to act in line with positive policies to prevent absence and encourage return to work. Good examples are available of the positive influence of vocational rehabilitation and linkage between health professionals and managers (Waddell et al, 2008). Small- and medium-sized employers may not have the capacity to offer these accommodations in the same way. Greater collaboration between policymakers with different agendas (such as the Department of Health and the Department for Work and Pensions in the UK) is crucial to support a change in culture and policy because it is not only the sick worker who will benefit from the new approach; there is growing evidence of the benefits for employers of efficient rehabilitation from employee health and wellbeing (PwC, 2009).

Potential implications of evolving models of management for older adults with musculoskeletal conditions

This new direction for managing musculoskeletal disorders and work participation in the United Kingdom (which has previously dealt with work absence only as an issue for the state doctor with provision for compensation) provides a model similar to that in North America in relation to workers' compensation (where there is greater employer involvement and a push to reduce absenteeism and improve worker performance). The objectives of these models are to aid sustained participation in work or return to work, and to direct a work-focused approach to patient care. Linking with the purpose of the new approach, empirical work from North America and the Fit for Work pilot studies provide examples of how consultations can become routinely work-focused and reduce absenteeism. However, these models will inevitably result in more presenteeism, that is, more people will continue to work despite having symptomatic musculoskeletal disorders, unable to complete important tasks in their job. What will then be the impact on performance and productivity, and cost to employers? These are key issues that must be addressed, because the impact of this new approach may fail if older workers with musculoskeletal disorders remain in the workplace with reduced productivity and place potential economic burdens on employers. The danger is that, as a consequence, employment rates of older workers with musculoskeletal disorders may decrease.

The need for further research

Despite much interest, there is relatively little research on the unique work issues of older adults with musculoskeletal disorders. The causes and consequences of work disability in older workers with musculoskeletal conditions, as discussed earlier, are complex, and may differ from those in younger workers. These need to be further explored to fully understand the implications of policy changes to working life, and to explore potential interventions to reduce adverse consequences of these changes. There is a need to identify the range of policy and research issues regarding health and safety issues of older workers that should be addressed over the coming decade. Building on the established foundations, consideration of the following issues may be useful to maintain the current momentum to improve work participation for those with musculoskeletal disorders.

How big is the problem? Epidemiology of musculoskeletal problems and work

Understanding future population trends, the potential demand for public services and costs will direct future planning. Projections of the size and structure of the older adult (50 years and over) workforce over the next 50 years would be useful to guide this. There is also a need to identify the groups that are more likely to have musculoskeletal disorders and work problems. The characteristics of work and older adults are evolving – the implications of this are unknown. Work is linked to the onset of some musculoskeletal conditions, and although work is becoming less physically demanding, this does not necessarily mean a reduction in incidence or prevalence; low back pain, for example, is common among workers in sedentary occupations (Garg and Moore, 1992). With changing characteristics, it would also be useful to identify tasks that are best suited to older adults to allow them to remain productive and in work. This may include a life-course approach. How does work change for an individual as he/she gets older? What are the key factors that influence work participation with age?

How should we measure work outcomes in older adults with musculoskeletal pain? Development of meaningful work outcomes

This depends on who is doing the measuring and here are some suggestions.

Clinicians

The frequency of musculoskeletal conditions means that work, in the form of return-to-work or work capacity, should be the outcome measure of choice for the management of musculoskeletal conditions in working-age adults. Work capacity/limitation can give a sense of an individual's ability to be productive on the job and meet essential job requirements. However, measurement of this is proving difficult. Standardised ways of measuring work capacity assume that individuals do not alter or modify their working practice. This may underestimate limitation due to the impact of accommodations in maintaining work capacity (Shaw and Feuerstein, 2004). Capacity is linked to performance and productivity, but what is the best way of measuring this? Most measures of performance and productivity are subjective; what does a subjective measure of performance mean? How does an individual's subjective view of their own performance link with that of their employer or objective data (Burton et al, 2010)? There is a need to develop the measurement of performance and productivity in a way that is acceptable to both clinicians and employers and would aid a common understanding of presenteeism. This would also help the development of a combined approach, through interaction of health and workplace interventions, to improve capacity and performance in adults with musculoskeletal conditions.

Policymakers

The policies that direct extensions to working life assume that older adults are able to continue to work for longer. However, if extensions in working life are accompanied by an increase in the period spent with musculoskeletal disorders and work disability, such targets will be difficult to realise and evidence to inform changes to pension age is essential. Measuring the number of years in good health and work is crucial to understanding the policy implications of extending working lives. Population health indicators (such as healthy life expectancy) have been developed to assess whether gains in life expectancy are years of healthy or unhealthy life. Healthy Working Life Expectancy (Lievre et al, 2007) is a longevity statistic that captures the number of years an average person of a particular age can expect to be both working and healthy. It is derived by combining data on health and employment status. Such an indicator may help to inform, guide and direct further research on work in older adults and the success of proposed interventions to maintain older workers in work.

Strategies and interventions

There is a lack of good-quality evidence to guide the preventive, therapeutic and rehabilitative arms of the response to the whole problem of musculoskeletal disorders and work (Walker-Bone and Cooper, 2005). This is important for practice needs. The starting point is to explore the predictors of work problems and build on the existing knowledge around work capability in older adults with musculoskeletal disorders. There has been limited work on older workers who have lower physical and mental capabilities to younger colleagues, and the few studies of transitions in work have not been detailed investigations of the mediating or moderating effects of co-morbidity, psychological and occupational factors (for example, Choi and Schlichting-Ray, 2001). This requires exploration of the complex interaction between musculoskeletal disorders, co-morbidities, psychological and occupational factors. It also requires consideration of the role of healthcare. This underpins a biopsychosocial approach to managing musculoskeletal conditions, and requires multidisciplinary and multicentre studies to fully understand how these factors interact will involve collaboration between researchers from different backgrounds, for example, occupational psychologists and sociologists, agencies and workers, and healthcare professionals.

An understanding of the mechanisms that dictate how long older adults remain in health and in work will inform current thinking about, and capture the feasibility and potential future success of, health practice aimed at extending working lives. By understanding the mechanisms by which physical, psychological, occupational and healthcare factors influence health and work in older workers with musculoskeletal disorders, better targeted interventions can be developed. This will be of considerable interest to public policy and health and social care professionals. Prevention will need to target both the impact of the musculoskeletal disorder and work disability. Current models of care to reduce the impact of musculoskeletal disorders on work will need to move towards more proactive preventive health policies related to the workplace, in similar ways to those that have emerged in primary care, which has moved from exclusive concern with sickness to being concerned with prevention of disease and reduction of disability through health promotion and screening programmes. This requires a shift towards promoting health in the worker and in the workplace as distinct from an exclusive concern with avoiding injury or dealing with sickness when it arises.

Following this, there is a need to explore the cost-effectiveness of accommodations and support programmes in the workplace and the community that can maintain work participation. Timing of interventions is important; although we know that being off work for a longer period increases the risk of long-term absence, more information is needed about the timing of interventions to ensure optimal outcomes. Much is known about ergonomic factors and the role of types of work and workplace environment in predisposing to musculoskeletal disorders, but there are many unanswered questions about prevention, causation, treatment and prognosis that must be addressed to ensure that the needs of those in work are being met.

As discussed previously, line managers are an important source of support in the workplace and play a mediating role within organisations. This role may be especially prominent in managing sustained participation in work and return to work for employees with musculoskeletal disorders. If line managers (for this we will focus on those on the front line who have direct contact with employees) are deficient in relevant skills and knowledge in advising and supporting people with these conditions, there may be barriers to return to work and excessive work loss. In this context, clarifying and developing the role of line managers may be an important means of promoting a healthy workforce.

The impact of staying in work for those with musculoskeletal disorders

In general, work is deemed to be good for health (Waddell and Burton, 2006), but further research is required to assess if this is true for all older workers who have musculoskeletal disorders. There has been little attention to the health and safety needs of older workers and there is a need to explore this. How will extensions to working life affect musculoskeletal disorders? Will this exacerbate their development? What will be the impact of prolonged working life on future health and wellbeing? What are the best methods to maximise opportunities for making employment-related choices that promote health, safety and life satisfaction in later years? If staying in work exacerbates musculoskeletal disorders, what is the additional cost to society in terms of health and social care costs? Investigation of the health and economic impact is required to provide further direction for policy on older workers.

Conclusion

The level of interest in musculoskeletal disorders and work is vital to continue to reduce the burden. Policies should continue to target improving work participation for people with musculoskeletal conditions to reduce the sizeable cost lost in lost productivity and sickness benefits. A national clinical director for musculoskeletal services could gather momentum and help services develop with the work agenda in mind. The introduction of the fit note should be viewed as a starting point to increase the biopsychosocial and interdisciplinary approach to managing musculoskeletal disorders and work. Further progress is challenging and evidence is needed to underpin this. Multidisciplinary and multicentre studies are needed to explore barriers to work participation and to evaluate future interventions that involve interaction between healthcare professionals and employers. Working with researchers in occupational psychology and sociology, as well as with agencies and workers themselves, will help healthcare professionals to plan future research and enhance work participation for people with musculoskeletal conditions. Local and systematic interventions in other countries have successfully improved outcomes for such patients and many of these principles can be adapted for the UK. The challenge has only just begun and we must continue to grasp the opportunities that arise.

Note

[1] www.dwp.gov.uk/health-work-and-well-being/our-work/fit-for-work-services.

Further reading

Bejarano, V., Quinn, M. and Conaghan, P.G. (2008) 'Effect of the early use of the anti-tumor necrosis factor adalimumab on the prevention of job loss in patients with early rheumatoid arthritis', *Arthritis Rheum*, vol 59, pp 1467-74.

Franche, R.L., Cullen, K., Clarke, J., Irvin, E., Sinclair, S. and Frank, J. (2005) 'Institute for Work & Health (IWH) Workplace-Based RTW Intervention Literature Review Research Team. Workplace-based return-to-work interventions: a systematic review of the quantitative literature', *Journal of Occupational Rehabilitation*, vol 15, pp 607-31.

Main, C.J., Sullivan, M.J.L. and Watson, P.J. (2007) *Pain management* (2nd edn), Edinburgh: Churchill Livingstone.

Waddell, G. (2006) 'Preventing incapacity in people with musculoskeletal disorders', *British Medical Bulletin*, vol 77-78, pp 55-69

WHO (World Health Organization) (2003) The burden of musculoskeletal conditions at the start of the new millennium: Report of a WHO scientific group, WHO Technical Report Series 919), Geneva: WHO.

References

Allaire, S. and Keysor, J.J. (2009) 'Development of a structured interview tool to help patients identify and solve rheumatic condition-related work barriers', *Arthritis Care & Research*, vol 61, no 7, pp 988-95.

Anis, A., Zhang, W., Emery, P., Sun, H., Singh, A., Freundlich, B. and Sato, R. (2009) 'The effect of etanercept on work productivity in patients with early active rheumatoid arthritis: results from the COMET study', *Rheumatology*, vol 48, no 10, pp 1283-9.

Bejarano, V., Quinn, M. and Conaghan, P.G. (2008) 'Effect of the early use of the anti-tumor necrosis factor adalimumab on the prevention of job loss in patients with early rheumatoid arthritis', *Arthritis Rheum*, vol 59, pp 1467-74.

Black, C. (2008) *Working for a healthier tomorrow*, London: The Stationery Office.

Boorman, S. (2009) www.nhshealthandwellbeing.org/FinalReport. html

Burton, W.N., Schultz, A., Chin, C.Y. and Edington, D.W. (2010) 'Work-associated arthritis productivity loss: where do we stand in its measurement?', *Journal of Rheumatology*, vol 37, pp 1792-3.

Campbell, J., Wright, C., Moseley, A., Chilvers, R., Richards, S. and Stabb, L. (2008) 'Avoiding long-term incapacity for work: Developing an early intervention in primary care', www.workingforhealth.gov.uk/ documents/developing-an-early-intervention-in-primary-care.pdf.

Choi, N.G. and Schlichting-Ray, L. (2001) 'Predictors of transitions in disease and disability in pre- and early-retirement populations', *Journal of Aging and Health*, vol 13, pp 379-409.

Cooper, C. 'New Med 3 "fit note" could be a breath of fresh air', http://community.healthcarerepublic.com/blogs/editors_blog/ archive/2010/02/01/new-med-3-fit-note-could-be-a-breath-of- fresh-air.aspx

Croft, P.R., Macfarlane, G.J., Papageorgiou, A.C., Thomas, E. and Silman, A.J. (1998) 'The outcome of low back pain in general practice: a prospective study', *British Medical Journal*, vol 316, pp 1356-9.

Currie, S.R. and Wang, J.L. (2004) 'Chronic back pain and major depression in the general Canadian population', *Pain*, vol 107, pp 54-60.

Druss, B.G., Rosenheck, R.A. and Sledge, W.H. (2000) 'Health and disability costs of depressive illness in a major US corporation', *American Journal of Psychiatry*, vol 157, pp 1274-8.

Dunn, K.M. and Croft, P.R. (2005) 'Classification of low back pain in primary care: using "bothersomeness" to identify the most severe cases', *Spine*, vol 30, pp 1887-92.

DWP (Department for Work and Pensions) and DH (Department of Health) (2008) *Improving health and work: Changing lives. The government's response to Dame Carol Black's review of the health of Britain's working-age population?* London: The Stationery Office.

Franche, R.L., Cullen, K., Clarke, J., Irvin, E., Sinclair, S. and Frank, J. (2005) 'Institute for Work & Health (IWH) Workplace-Based RTW Intervention Literature Review Research Team. Workplace-based return-to-work interventions: a systematic review of the quantitative literature', *Journal of Occupational Rehabilitation*, vol 15, pp 607-31.

Garg, A. and Moore, J.S. (1992) 'Epidemiology of low-back pain in industry', *Occupational Medicine*, vol 7, pp 593-608.

Gilworth, G., Chamberlain, M.A., Harvey, A., Woodhouse, A., Smith, J., Smyth, M.G. and Tennant, A. (2003) 'Development of a work instability scale for rheumatoid arthritis', *Arthritis Rheum*, vol 49, pp 349-54.

Hestbaek, L., Leboeuf, Y.C. and Manniche, C. (2003) 'Low back pain: what is the long-term course? A review of studies of general patient populations', *European Spine Journal, vol* **12**, pp 149-65.

Holdsworth, L.K., Webster, V. and McFadyen, A.K. (2007) 'What are the costs to NHS Scotland of self-referral to physiotherapy? Results of a national trial', *Physiotherapy*, vol 93, pp 3-11.

Jinks, C., Jordan, K., Ong, B.N. and Croft, P. (2004) 'A brief screening tool for knee pain in primary care (KNEST). 2. Results from a survey in the general population aged 50 and over', *Rheumatology*, vol 43, pp 55-61.

Jinks, C., Jordan, K.P. and Croft, P. (2007) 'Osteoarthritis as a public health problem: the impact of developing knee pain on physical function in adults living in the community: (KNEST 3)', *Rheumatology*, vol 46, pp 877-81.

Lee, M.C. and Tracey, I. (2010) 'Unravelling the mystery of pain, suffering, and relief with brain imaging', *Current Pain and Headache Reports*, vol 14, pp 124-31.

Lerner, D., Amick, B.C. 3rd, Rogers, W.H., Malspeis, S., Bungay, K. and Cynn, D. (2001) 'The Work Limitations Questionnaire', *Medical Care*, vol 39, pp 72-85.

Lievre, A., Jusot, F., Barnay, T., Sermet, C., Brouard, N., Robine, J.M., Brieu, M.A. and Forette, F. (2007) 'Healthy working life expectancies at age 50 in Europe: a new indicator', *Journal of Nutrition, Health and Aging*, vol 11, no 6, pp 508-14.

Linton, S.J. and Andersson, T. (2000) 'Can chronic disability be prevented? A randomized trial of a cognitive-behavior intervention and two forms of information for patients with spinal pain', *Spine*, vol 25, pp 2825-31.

Main, C.J., Sullivan, M.J.L. and Watson, P.J. (2007) *Pain Management* (2nd edn), Edinburgh: Churchill Livingstone.

Maniadakis, N. and Gray, A. (2000) 'The economic burden of back pain in the UK', *Pain*, vol 84, pp 95-103.

Marmot, M., Allen, J., Goldblatt, P., Boyce, T., McNeish, D., Grady, M. and Geddes, I. (2010) *Fair society, healthy lives: The Marmot review, strategic review of health inequalities in England post-2010*. London: Department of Health.

NAO (National Audit Office) (2009) *Services for people with rheumatoid arthritis*, London: The Stationery Office.

National Rheumatoid Arthritis Society (2003) *'Beyond the pain'; The social and psychological impact of RA.* Maidenhead: National Rheumatoid Arthritis Society.

Pransky, G., Shaw, W., Franche, R.L. and Clarke, A. (2004) 'Disability prevention and communication among workers, physicians, employers, and insurers – current models and opportunities for improvement', *Disability and Rehabilitation*, vol 26, no 11, pp 625-34.

PwC (PricewaterhouseCoopers) (2008) 'Building the case for wellness', www.workingforhealth.gov.uk/documents/dwp-wellness-report-public.pdf.

Sanders, C., Donovan, J.L. and Dieppe, P.A. (2004) 'Unmet need for joint replacement: a qualitative investigation of barriers to treatment among individuals with severe pain and disability of the hip and knee', *Rheumatology*, vol 43, no 3, pp 353-7.

Shaw, W.S. and Feuerstein, M. (2004) 'Generating workplace accommodations: lessons learned from the integrated case management study', *Journal of Occupational Rehabilitation*, vol 14, no 3, pp 207-16.

Shaw, W.S., Means-Christensen, A., Slater, M.A., Patterson, T.L., Webster, J.S. and Atkinson, J.H. (2007) 'Shared and independent associations of psychosocial factors on work status among men with subacute low back pain', *Clinical Journal of Pain*, vol 23, pp 409-16.

Shaw, W.S., Pransky, G. and Winters, T. (2009) 'The Back Disability Risk Questionnaire for work-related, acute back pain: prediction of unresolved problems at 3-month follow-up', *Journal of Occupational Environmental Medicine*, vol 51, pp 185-94.

Sullivan, M.J.L., Adams, H., Tripp, D. and Stanish, W.D. (2008) 'Stage of chronicity and treatment response in patients with musculoskeletal injuries and concurrent symptoms of depression', *Pain*, vol 135, pp 151-9.

Symmons, D., Tunrer, G., Webb, R., Asten, P., Barrett, E., Lunt, M., Scott, D. and Silman, A. (2002) 'The prevalence of rheumatoid arthritis in the United Kingdom: new estimates for a new century', *Rheumatology*, vol 41, no 7, pp 793-800.

Thomas, E., Peat, G., Harris, L., Wilkie, R. and Croft, P.R. (2004) 'The prevalence of pain and pain interference in a general population of older adults: cross-sectional findings from the North Staffordshire Osteoarthritis Project (NorStOP)', *Pain*, vol 110, pp 361-8.

Waddell, G. (2006) 'Preventing incapacity in people with musculoskeletal disorders', *British Medical Bulletin*, vol 77-78, pp 55-69.

Waddell, G. and Burton, A.K. (2006) *Is work good for your health and well-being?*, London: The Stationery Office.

Waddell, G., Burton, A.K. and Kendall, N.A.S. (2008) *Vocational rehabilitation: What works, for whom, and when?*, London: The Stationery Office.

Walker-Bone, K. and Cooper, C. (2005) 'Hard work never hurt anyone: or did it? A review of occupational associations with soft tissue musculoskeletal disorders of the neck and upper limb', *Annals of Rheumatic Diseases*, vol 64, no 10, pp 1391-6.

WHO (World Health Organization) (2003) *The burden of musculoskeletal conditions at the start of the new millennium: Report of a WHO scientific group*, WHO Technical Report Series 919, Geneva: WHO.

Williamson, G.M. and Schulz, R. (1992) 'Pain, activity restriction, and symptoms of depression among community-residing elderly adults', *Journal of Gerontology*, vol 47, no 14, pp 367-72.

Woolf, A.D. (2000) 'The bone and joint decade 2000-2010', *Annals of Rheumatic Diseases*, vol 59, pp 81-2

Woolf, D. and Pfleger, D. (2003) 'Burden of major musculoskeletal conditions', *Bulletin of the World Health Organization*, vol 81, p 9.

Young, A., Dixey, J., Cox, N., Davies, P., Devlin, J., Emery, P., Gallivan, S., Gough, A., James, D., Prouse, P., Williams, P. and Winfield, J. (2005) 'How does functional disability in early rheumatoid (RA) affect patients and their lives? Results of 5 years of follow up in 732 patients from the Early RA Study (ERAS)', *Rheumatology*, vol 39, pp 603-11.

THREE

Common mental health problems and work

Annie Irvine

Introduction

Recent years have seen significant policy attention focused on mental health and employment. The latter part of 2009 saw the publication of several key documents, including the first national strategy on mental health and employment (Health, Work and Wellbeing Directorate, 2009), an overarching framework for mental health service provision (HM Government, 2009a), a review of support for people not in employment due to mental health conditions (DWP, 2009), a strategy on employment support for people in contact with secondary mental health services (HM Government, 2009b) and public health guidelines for line managers on creating mentally healthy workplaces (NICE, 2009). Preceding these reports, Dame Carol Black's 2008 review of the health of the working-age population drew particular attention to the prevalence of mental ill health and its substantial impact on absenteeism and worklessness (Black, 2008; Lelliott et al, 2008).

This suite of publications covers a diverse range of economic and social concerns, from supporting the employment of people who experience severe mental health conditions, through reducing the incapacity benefits bill (the largest proportion of which is attributable to mental ill health), to the promotion of positive mental wellbeing among the whole workforce. In a chapter of this size it is only possible to focus on a few of these areas. The present discussion will concentrate on the retention of paid employment, rather than transitions into work from unemployment[1] and the main focus will be on what are known as *mild to moderate* or *common* mental health problems. These terms are generally used to denote a range of anxiety conditions and less severe forms of depression that 'cause marked emotional distress and interfere with daily function, but do not usually affect insight or cognition' (Deverill and King, 2009, p 25). While not currently a diagnostic category in itself, work-related stress is often discussed in the same context. For example, Waddell and Burton (2006, p 22) state that stress 'may be the best modern exemplar of common mental health problems', while a report for the mental health charity Mind (Robertson, 2005, p 7) considers that 'stress at work is now one of the most common forms of mental distress'.

Common mental health problems are thought to affect around one in six of the adult population of Britain (Singleton et al, 2001; Deverill and King, 2009). For both men and women, symptoms of a severity likely to require treatment are most prevalent among those aged 45-54. Survey evidence suggests that one quarter of women aged 45-54 meet diagnostic criteria for at least one common mental health problem (Deverill and King, 2009). While prevalence rates decrease quite sharply among the 55-64 age group for both genders, this suggests that 'younger' older workers are at particular risk of mental health problems, perhaps during the peak of their career.[2]

Taken together, work-related stress, depression and anxiety accounted for an estimated 11.4 million lost working days in 2008/09, affecting 415,000 people (HSE, 2010). Mirroring overall population prevalence rates, the 2008/09 Labour Force Survey found that reports of work-related stress, anxiety and depression were highest among the 45-54 age group. The combined costs to business of absenteeism, presenteeism[3] and staff turnover related to mental ill health total £26 billion per year or £1,035 per employee (CMH, 2007), while mental ill health costs the national economy an estimated £30-40 billion annually in sick pay, incapacity benefits and NHS treatment (Health, Work and Wellbeing Directorate, 2009). Thus, common mental health problems among the working-age population have a substantial financial impact on individual business and on the national economy.

There are also significant personal and social impacts at the micro level. Employees with experience of mental health problems report a range of problematic effects on their day-to-day work including poor concentration, difficulties with social interactions, fatigue (linked to disturbed sleep), agitation and physical side effects of medication (Honey, 2002; Haslam et al, 2005; Irvine, 2008; Sainsbury et al, 2008). All of these effects are challenging for the individual and may also have a direct impact on others at work, including line managers, colleagues and customers or clients. This combination of prevalence, economic and social impact makes the understanding of what helps to manage common mental health problems a key priority for policy and business.

However, mental health is a hugely complex field, encompassing a multitude of concepts, connotations, language and lived experience. There are still many unknowns about the origins or causes of mental health problems and while qualitative research consistently reports a perspective that work-related factors can 'trigger' or exacerbate mental health problems (for example, Thomas et al, 2003; Haslam et al, 2005; Irvine, 2008; Sainsbury et al, 2008; Coe, 2009; Pittam et al, 2010), common mental health problems frequently have their origins outside of the workplace. As such, there will always be factors that are beyond the immediate control of employers and 'however well managed a workplace is, it will contain people experiencing substantial levels of mental ill health' (Seymour, 2010a, p 59).

This complexity makes establishing 'what works' to reduce the impact of mental health problems at work a particularly challenging task. This chapter outlines the current knowledge base about what helps in managing common mental health problems at work along with consideration of the context-dependent nature of outcomes and some suggested future research directions. Before this, however, the following section introduces some key conceptual and theoretical questions, drawing particular attention to notions of mental health as a continuum and as a fluctuating state of being. While it is beyond the scope of this chapter to fully explore these debates, there are some important ways in which they may have a bearing on approaches to managing common mental health problems at work, and so they are important to acknowledge.

Mental health: what are we talking about?

A fundamental challenge when thinking about common mental health problems and work is establishing what it is that we are talking about. As noted earlier, common mental health problems are typically taken to include anxiety and depression but may also be deemed to include work-related stress. Recently, policy attention has also turned towards *mental wellbeing* as a public health issue, with mental health referred to as something to be proactively promoted and protected. Here, we find the notion that a person might experience poor mental health without necessarily having a clinically significant mental health condition, but that the former might lead to the latter (Health, Work and Wellbeing Directorate, 2009; HM Government, 2009a). Some scholars suggest that mental distress and wellbeing are positioned along a single continuum (for example, Wilson and Beresford, 2002), while others consider the possibility of distinct (though related) dimensions of mental health, mental distress and mental disorder (Payton, 2009; Westerhof and Keyes, 2010). Horwitz (2007, p 285) asserts that we should 'distinguish the proportionate responses of distressed people to stressful social arrangements from the psychological disorders that these arrangements can sometimes produce'.[4] Common mental health problems thus occupy a contested position between concepts of poor mental wellbeing, stress, distress and clinically significant 'disorder'.

To some extent, it might be argued that these nuanced theoretical debates are of secondary importance, given the significant material impact of stress on the workplace. The presence or absence of a clinical diagnosis will not necessarily determine the nature of an individual's experience or its impact on work. Whether badged as work-related stress, anxiety, depression, emotional exhaustion or burnout, these combined experiences of psychological distress have a significant and detrimental effect on workplace productivity and the personal lives of those concerned.

However, there are ways in which conceptualisations of poor mental health as stress, distress or illness may have significance when considering the management of mental health and work, with regard to disclosure, help seeking and support. For example, notwithstanding the well-documented concerns about stigma and discrimination, when it comes to common mental health problems 'disclosure may not occur simply because the individual does not consider that their current experience constitutes a "mental health problem" to be disclosed' (Irvine, 2011). The Centre for Mental Health (CMH, 2007, p 6) similarly notes that 'in many cases clinically diagnosable mental health problems are not recognised or acknowledged as such even by the individuals directly affected'. There is also some evidence that employers perceive limits to their role and responsibilities in relation to 'personal' problems (Rolfe et al, 2006) and that line managers may be unresponsive to non-medicalised expressions of distress (Irvine, 2011). Attempts at early intervention may thus be hampered by a lack of recognition or engagement before such time as problems become acute. This is an issue recognised in the National Strategy for Mental Health and Employment:

> Employees should feel enabled to discuss potential issues with their managers before distress becomes prolonged or serious enough to impede performance at work or lead to absence. This is true even where the cause of distress is something that has happened outside the workplace. (Health, Work and Wellbeing Directorate, 2009, p 30)

Linked to notions of mental health as a continuum, it is important to recognise that mental health can fluctuate. Regardless of whether we perceive a single continuum of mental health and ill health, or separate dimensions of wellbeing and distress, it is clear that for most people, the experience of mental health problems is not continuous or static in nature. Difficulties may recur over time, but there will often be long periods where mental health is not acutely or even significantly problematic to the individual. Some people who experience recurrent periods of anxiety or depression may choose to adopt a notion of 'recovery' whereby they see themselves as managing a long-term condition. However, others may consider their experiences as short term or 'one off' and not consider themselves to 'have' a mental health condition at all once symptoms have ameliorated.

Perhaps unavoidably, the language used in policy publications tends to be simplified to 'people *with* mental health conditions' or 'people *who have* mental health conditions', both of which imply a degree of permanent clinical significance that seems at odds with a notion of mental health as a fluctuating continuum. For example, the National Strategy (Health, Work and Wellbeing Directorate, 2009) explicitly sets out a 'dual approach', addressing on the one hand employment support and improved outcomes for 'people with mental health conditions' and other the other hand improved wellbeing at work for 'everyone'. But when thinking about common mental health problems among workers, it is important to recognise that we are not referring to a discrete or homogenous group of people who have a clear-cut, stable or permanent 'condition' of mental ill health. Consider, for example, a person who has, at some point in their life, crossed the threshold into meeting diagnostic criteria for depression or an anxiety disorder but who has, through a combination of effective strategies, recovered to the point at which they no longer meet clinical thresholds. Nevertheless, they continue to implement such strategies in order to stay well. Is this person still managing a mental health 'condition' or are they now simply taking care of their mental wellbeing? What is their status and where do they fit within current policy?

The conceptual issues outlined above also pose challenges in thinking through what it means to 'manage mental health and work'. If mental health is a continuum along which anyone might move at different times in response to life circumstances, it is perhaps an artificial distinction to talk separately of prevention and management of mental health problems. As will be noted, there is a substantial degree of overlap in the strategies that may be useful in each of these respects. However, for the present purposes, we focus on strategies that might help to minimise the impact of common mental health problems at work when they occur.

What helps to manage common mental health problems at work?

Recent systematic reviews on what interventions are effective in helping people to manage common mental health problems at work include Seymour and Grove (2005), Hill and colleagues (2007), Underwood and colleagues (2007), Waddell and colleagues (2008) and Seymour (2010b). All have found that the evidence base is small, particularly for UK-based studies (Seymour, 2010b), and with results often inconclusive (Underwood et al, 2007).[5] However, the specific focus on 'interventions' may in part account for the small amount of evidence identified by systematic reviews. For example, while Underwood et al (2007, p 6) state that they took a very broad definition of what constituted an intervention, they acknowledge the possibility that their review revealed few studies 'because there are few interventions; people with common mental health problems may simply be given medication and not offered any further support' (p 9). Alongside studies meeting the criteria for inclusion in systematic reviews, there is also a modest amount of 'softer' evidence from survey and qualitative research that describes a quite consistent range of factors that people find helpful (or unhelpful) in remaining in or returning to work in the context of common mental health problems (for example, Thomas et al, 2003; Depression Alliance, 2008; Irvine, 2008; Sainsbury et al, 2008).

When employees experience common mental health problems, there are a number of aspects to be addressed in reducing the impact on work, including minimising the impact on attendance and productivity, minimising the duration of necessary absences and supporting reintegration to the workplace following absence. Qualitative research with people who have experience of managing common mental health problems in work (Irvine, 2008) suggests that, to a large extent, similar strategies are useful in each of these respects. They include flexibility and workplace adjustments; employer awareness and engagement; access to effective medical treatment; and strategies for keeping well in the longer term. The role of vocational rehabilitation services has also been emphasised in recent review evidence (Seymour, 2010b). The next section considers each of these themes alongside recent policy that responds or corresponds to each.

Flexibility and workplace adjustments

Flexibility emerges as central to managing work alongside the experience of common mental health problems (for example, Gray,

1999; Depression Alliance, 2008; Irvine, 2008). Useful types of flexibility may pertain to the number of hours worked in a given day or week, the specific hours worked or the location of work, for example, being able to work from home either on a permanent or occasional basis. These flexibilities might be used responsively, for example, working from home during periods of more severe anxiety or depression, or pre-emptively, for example, using flexitime to avoid rush-hour commuting or deliberately accruing time off in lieu in order to take rest days at regular intervals. Both approaches may be helpful in avoiding the need for repeated or prolonged periods of sickness absence (Irvine, 2008). The ability to take time off during the working day to attend medical appointments or therapy sessions may also be appreciated. Further adjustments that individuals may find useful include quiet rooms to work in or 'time out' spaces, more frequent breaks, changes in role to remove tasks that cause anxiety and more regular support from supervisors (Gray, 1999; Irvine, 2008; DWP, 2009).

The Equality Act 2010 places a duty on employers to make 'reasonable adjustments' for employees who have a mental or physical disability and the DWP-administered Access to Work fund may be available to assist with implementing workplace adjustments. The 2008 green paper *No one written off* (DWP, 2008) called for suggestions as to how this fund could be used more effectively with respect to mental health problems, while a recent pilot project in two areas of London, funded by Access to Work, has reported positive outcomes for its clients.[6] The Perkins review (DWP, 2009) made the important observation that it is often the social world of work, rather than the physical environment, that is most difficult to negotiate for a person experiencing a mental health condition: 'The adjustments required tend therefore to centre on workplace social interactions and relationships with support required not only by the individual but also their managers/employers and colleagues' (DWP, 2009, p 29). As such, the kinds of adjustment found useful in relation to common mental health problems may not require financial investment, but may require a willingness to be flexible and responsive to individual needs.

Employer awareness and engagement

Line managers are considered to be central to the effective management of work and mental health. Their understanding of mental health problems, ability to recognise distress among their staff and confidence to intervene early and sensitively may be influential on work outcomes (Irvine, 2008; Sainsbury et al, 2008). A number of guidance documents have been produced aimed at line managers, including the 'Line manager's resource' produced by the cross-governmental Shift Action on Stigma campaign[7] and 'Taking care of business' produced by Mind as part of its 2010 campaign on workplace mental health.[8] During 2008, the Centre for Mental Health piloted Impact on Depression, a workplace mental health programme targeted at line managers. Based on a proven Australian model,[9] the programme aims to 'build the knowledge, confidence and skills of managers and staff, in supporting people with depression and other mental health conditions to access timely treatment that can promote their recovery while in work' (Seymour, 2010b, p 8). Evaluation of the UK pilot indicated positive changes in line managers' knowledge, attitudes and confidence to engage with employees experiencing common mental health problems.[10]

Another employer-focused initiative is the Mindful Employer programme,[11] which aims to increase awareness of mental ill health and provide information and support for employers in the recruitment and retention of staff. Mindful Employer offers information, resources, signposting, peer support, training and practical support. More generally, positive workplace relationships can be a key factor in supporting an individual to remain in work during times of mental ill health and can be an encouragement to return to work from absence (Irvine, 2008).

Access to effective medical treatment

There is substantial evidence that psychological therapy is effective in alleviating the symptoms of common mental health problems. Government is investing in evidence-based 'talking therapies' through the Improving Access to Psychological Therapies (IAPT) programme.[12] IAPT aims to increase capacity to treat depression and anxiety by training an additional 3,600 psychological therapists in the delivery of NICE-approved treatments (DH, 2010). Cognitive behavioural therapy (CBT) is currently held to be one of the most effective approaches for mild to moderate anxiety and depression, and forms the core component of the IAPT offer. However, CBT is not without critics (see Leach, 2009, p 11) and the policy intention is to offer a wider choice of evidence-based treatment as the programme expands (DH, 2010). The two original IAPT demonstration sites are being evaluated by the University of Sheffield with results due to be published in late 2010. While there is currently some dispute about the effectiveness of anti-depressant drugs for more moderate forms of depression (for example, Fournier et al, 2010), prescribed medications are also reported to be helpful by some people, either as a short-term or longer-term management strategy (Irvine, 2008).

Vocational rehabilitation services

The importance of vocational rehabilitation services for employees experiencing common mental health problems has recently been emphasised (Waddell et al, 2008; Seymour, 2010b). These services offer independent case management, providing 'a skilled brokerage function to act for the employee and as an intermediary with other critical partners in health and employment' (Seymour, 2010a, p 60). Provision of such services in the UK is currently said to be 'patchy and poorly funded' (Boyce et al, 2009, p 23). However, policy recognition of the potential of job retention services can be found in the Fit for Work Services currently being piloted in 11 locations across the UK. These services focus on early intervention to limit the duration of sickness absence and are expected to take a coordinated and holistic approach to addressing health, employment and wider social support needs (such as housing or debt). Employment advisers have also been placed within IAPT teams, working alongside therapists to provide advice and support to help people remain in or make a quicker return to work.[13]

A small-scale qualitative evaluation of a recent initiative in the south of England found positive outcomes for people seeking to retain work (Pittam et al, 2010). In particular, clients of this service benefited from careers guidance, developing strategies to negotiate and communicate with employers and assistance to think about the potential benefits of a career change. Positive outcomes were also experienced by most participants in another small-scale pilot reported by Thomas and colleagues (2003). However, findings from a randomised controlled trial conducted in the UK (Purdon et al, 2006) found that people on mental health-related absence from work who had received service intervention had a lower likelihood of returning to work than those who did not. Further analysis (Taylor and Lewis, 2008) suggested that explanations for delayed return to work among this group included waiting for a more complete health recovery, dependency on the provider, or the fact that seeking a new job may have been more productive than focusing on returning to the same employer. Also, there seemed to be less scope to boost NHS provision for mental health as compared with other conditions and less scope to improve the workplace context beyond that which (supportive) employers were already willing to provide.

Strategies for keeping well

For people who have had experience of common mental health problems, steps to maintain better mental health in the longer term may be important in reducing the risk of recurrence. Qualitative research with people who had past or ongoing experience of common mental health problems (Irvine, 2008) indicated that a number of strategies could be important in maintaining positive mental health. Alongside flexible working arrangements (as noted earlier), a key strategy was effective stress management and good 'work–life balance'. Other factors that helped people to stay well included maintaining physical health and good nutrition, positive workplace relationships, work itself (where suitable and enjoyable), supportive friendships and family relationships, relaxation, spiritual engagement and a growing understanding of personal 'triggers' or warning signs.

It is notable that many of these strategies mirror current advice on how to promote mental wellbeing. Individual behaviours that are perceived to protect against mental health problems and strengthen mental wellbeing, and may in turn increase resilience in times of difficulty, include such things as keeping physically fit, eating well, taking time to relax, learning and being creative, maintaining social networks and taking part in voluntary and community activities (Friedli et al, 2007; Foresight Mental Capital and Wellbeing Project, 2008; Mental Health Foundation, 2008). The parallel messages about what helps to prevent both the occurrence and the recurrence of mental health problems brings us back to the notion of mental health as a continuum and suggests that the management of mental health is perhaps a long-term project in which each and all of us are engaged.

Discussion: the key role of context

The previous sections have presented a number of factors that might help to minimise the impact of common mental health problems at work. However, at the individual level there are few certainties or clear-cut answers. The impact of mental health problems on employment outcomes will depend on the nature and interplay of a wide range of work and non-work factors.

A particularly important finding to emerge from recent research is that effective intervention for people experiencing common mental health problems requires a dual approach, focusing both on clinical and vocational support. While medication and psychological treatment can be beneficial in reducing symptoms, used alone, they do not necessarily improve work outcomes (Sanderson and Andrews, 2006; Lelliott et al, 2008; Waddell et al, 2008; Seymour, 2010b). Common mental health problems do not exist in isolation of an individual's broader personal and social context. With regard to successful employment outcomes, the specific nature of an individual's work – including role, working environment and co-worker relationships – may be crucial. As summarised by Lelliott and colleagues (2008, p 39), 'The interactions between symptoms, work performance, sickness absence and return to work are complex and greatly influenced by contextual factors both in the individual and in the workplace'.

It is also important to remember that, while experiences of anxiety or depression are often problematic to a person's day-to-day work, this is not necessarily the case. While the cumulative economic impact of common mental health problems on workplaces is clear, many individuals are able to stay in work throughout periods of anxiety or depression without taking absence and with minimal impact on their productivity. The extent to which the individual enjoys their work, and gains satisfaction and fulfilment from it, is likely to play a part in their perception of whether work is compatible with periods of mental ill health (Irvine, 2008). For some people who perceive the origins of their distress to be outside of the workplace, coming to work may be experienced as a respite. Moreover, work may be a positive factor in alleviating mental health problems. As is now well recognised, good work is good for you (Waddell and Burton, 2006).

On the other hand, for some people, work may be perceived as unmanageable alongside the effort required to get well or to focus on addressing the non-work causes of mental distress. Moreover, the work-related nature of some mental health problems may pose particular challenges to job retention and effective employer support. Whether or not mental health problems are perceived to have been caused by work is likely to have a significant influence both on an individual's day-by-day decisions about being at work and on overall decisions about job retention. While prolonged lack of contact with the workplace increases the difficulty of making a return from absence, maintaining supportive and constructive dialogue may be difficult where negative workplace circumstances are perceived to have contributed to the development of problems:

> Not uncommonly, a position develops where an individual has recovered sufficiently to consider returning to work but perceives that exposure to his employers, colleagues or

other aspects of the work will lead to a relapse (Henderson et al, 2005, p 802).

Furthermore, whether or not contact with a line manager or colleagues is appreciated during periods of absence will vary among individuals and there may be challenges in achieving the right degree of input at times when an individual is most unwell. While early intervention is considered to be crucial to effective support of an employee experiencing mental health problems, employer involvement 'needs to be sensitively handled or the intervention may exacerbate the problem' (Gray, 1999, p 7).

Adjusting to changed capacity for work following the experience of anxiety or depression may also be challenging for the individual. Although the avoidance of stress is frequently noted as important, a job that is perceived as too undemanding may also exacerbate mental health problems. Balancing the desire for work that is in line with personal interests and intellect against the need to take on less stressful work that does not exacerbate mental health problems can be a difficult compromise where people feel frustrated that they are working below their potential (Honey, 2002; Irvine, 2008). This reinforces the potentially beneficial role of vocational rehabilitation services in assisting people in 'broadening their perspective regarding their future employment prospects' (Pittam et al, 2010, p 7).

This combination of individual, environmental and occupational factors means that it is difficult to generalise about what will help a given individual to stay in work during periods of mental ill health or to predict the impact on their work. However, it seems that the extent to which jobs allow the required degree of flexibility is central and that individual interests and preferences must be taken into account. In the field of occupational therapy, this has been referred to as the 'occupation competence model' (Shaw and Polatajko, 2002) or 'person-environment-occupation fit' (Law et al, 1996; Kirsh, 2000). These approaches recognise that the impact of health conditions on work is contextually bound and can only be understood through consideration of the person, the environment, the occupation and the interrelationships between these three dimensions (Shaw and Polatajko, 2002). Comparing two groups of individuals with long-term experience of severe mental health problems, Kirsh (2000) found that perceptions of person-environment fit were significantly higher among those who retained employment than those who had recently left their jobs.

An implication of this is that changing employers entirely may sometimes be the most appropriate way forward for someone who has experienced common mental health problems. While employers have a duty to offer reasonable adjustments, there may be situations where an individual concludes that a particular role is simply not right for them. The challenge then is to make as seamless a transition as possible, avoiding the risk of falling on to benefits from which the move back to work can be an even more challenging task.

Conclusion and future research directions

Research priorities recently identified by the Medical Research Council (MRC, 2010) focus on further understanding the biomedical and social determinants of mental ill health and on developing effective medicine and therapies to prevent or alleviate mental health problems. However, given the evidence that a focus on clinical treatments alone is unlikely to improve work outcomes, there is also a need for further research into what employment-focused interventions and support are most effective for people who are experiencing common mental health problems.

Among a number of important research gaps identified by Lelliott and colleagues (2008, p 44), one key question is about what features 'of a mental health problem, of the individual, of the work environment and of the context' make retention in or return to work difficult. Due to the individual and context-dependent nature of mental health experiences, it seems that qualitative approaches must be central to any further research attempts to uncover the complex range of influences that determine individual work outcomes. Following the example of Karp (1996), more phenomenological research into the lived experience of common mental health problems would also be valuable. Exploring individual perceptions of the causes and course of illness experience is important, because how mental health is understood has implications for how mental health problems are responded to, both by the individual and by others who have a potential role in providing support.

Another gap in understanding relates to the managers and colleagues of individuals experiencing common mental health problems. While attention is often drawn to their low levels of awareness and potential role in exacerbating mental health problems, little research to date has explored the first-hand experiences of line managers and co-workers in relation to supporting and working with a colleague during periods of anxiety, depression or stress-related illness (though see Rolfe et al, 2006 and Sainsbury et al, 2008). A key message of current policy on health and work is that it is not necessary to be completely well in order to be at work, with attempts to challenge the 'belief that we should always refrain from work when we have a health condition' (Health, Work and Wellbeing Directorate, 2008, p 10). However, while common mental health problems by no means preclude work, they do at times have an effect on the individual's day-to-day performance, which may in turn affect those around them. With the current policy aim to have more people *at work* while experiencing common mental health problems, it is important to know more about how this affects the workplace more broadly and what support may be needed by others who have a role in facilitating job retention.

Additionally, much of the research on experiences of managing mental health and work has been conducted within large organisations. There is currently a paucity of evidence on the impact of employee mental health problems on micro, small and medium enterprises, for whom the day-to-day impact of common mental health problems on co-workers and on overall productivity may be far more immediate and significant. Research exploring the capacity of small firms to respond to the requirements of the Equality Act (or its predecessor the Disability Discrimination Act) for employees with mental health problems, and the financial and practical impacts of doing so, is currently lacking (though see Goss and Goss, 1998). The National Institute for Health and Clinical Excellence (NICE, 2009) identifies a need for research on effective and cost effective models for the promotion of mental wellbeing in micro, small and medium-sized businesses. With most evidence currently coming from medium to large organisations, it is not yet clear whether the economic case for investment in mental health and wellbeing applies equally to micro and small businesses.

This chapter has sought to provide an overview of the current evidence base on managing common mental health problems at work and related policy responses. The fit of work with individual capacities and preferences, the need for flexibility and the role of workplace relations are all strongly implicated in retention, rehabilitation and staying well. Line managers have a key role to play, but there is growing evidence that input from independent vocational rehabilitation services may be important in brokering successful job retention. Crucially, successful management of mental health and work depends on much more than alleviating clinical symptoms. A focus on the mental health condition in isolation will often be insufficient because so much depends on the specific nature of the individual's employment and their wider personal and social circumstances. In sum, the experience of managing mental health and work is unique to each individual, and therein lies perhaps the biggest challenge.

Finally, alongside current evidence on effective strategies, this chapter has also attempted to highlight some of the more complex conceptual and theoretical debates about mental health that underlie this major area of policy concern and the challenges that they may entail. While it has only been possible to skim the surface of such debates, it is important to acknowledge the complexity that always underlies any more policy-oriented consideration of mental health and work. To overlook this complexity would hamper attempts to understand individual experiences and thereby to begin to understand 'what works'.

Notes

[1] While there is likely to be some overlap in which strategies are effective, it has been suggested that these different areas of concern require different approaches and should be addressed separately (Bacon et al, 2010; Boyce et al, 2009; Pittam et al, 2010).

[2] It should be noted that prevalence rates among males are fairly stable across the 25-54 age group, while for women the greater prevalence among 45-54 year olds is more marked (see Deverill and King, 2009, p 30).

[3] Defined as 'the loss in productivity that occurs when employees come to work but function at less than full capacity because of ill health' (CMH, 2007, p 3).

[4] It is also important to note the wider sociological debates that consider the role of institutions and culture in the construction of 'mental illness' and thereby call into question the fundamental validity or usefulness of diagnostic categories (see, for example, Bolton, 2007; Bowers, 1998).

[5] This is in notable contrast to the much larger amount of research evidence on severe mental health conditions and employment, despite such conditions being far less prevalent (Underwood et al, 2007).

[6] www.mind.org.uk/news/1465_mind_helps_pave_the_way_for_better_mental_health_support_at_work

[7] The Shift campaign formally comes to an end in 2010 and further hard copies of the resource will not be produced. At the time of writing, it was not clear whether the online resource would remain accessible.

[8] www.mind.org.uk/employment

[9] www.beyondblue.org.au

[10] www.centreformentalhealth.org.uk/pdfs/workplace_programme_intro.pdf

[11] www.mindfulemployer.net

[12] www.iapt.nhs.uk

[13] For details on Fit for Work Services and IAPT employment advisers, see www.workingforhealth.gov.uk/initatives

Further reading

Health, Work and Wellbeing Directorate (2009) *Working our way to better mental health: A framework for action*, Norwich: The Stationery Office, www.official-documents.gov.uk/document/cm77/7756/7756.pdf

Irvine, A. (2008) *Managing mental health and employment*, DWP Research Report 537, London: Department for Work and Pensions, available at http://research.dwp.gov.uk/asd/asd5/rports2007-2008/rrep537.pdf

Rolfe, H., Foreman, J. and Tylee, A. (2006) *Welfare of farewell? Mental health and stress in the workplace*, NIESR Discussion Paper 268, London: National Institute of Social and Economic Research, available at www.niesr.ac.uk/pdf/270306_133707.pdf

Sainsbury, R., Irvine, A., Aston, J., Wilson, S., Williams, C. and Sinclair, A. (2008) *Mental health and employment*, DWP Research Report 513, London: Department for Work and Pensions, available at http://research.dwp.gov.uk/asd/asd5/rports2007-2008/rrep513.pdf

Seymour, L. (2010b) *Common mental health problems at work. What we know about successful interventions. A progress review*, London: Centre for Mental Health, available at www.centreformentalhealth.org.uk/pdfs/BOHRF_common_mental_health_problems_at_work.pdf

References

Bacon, J., Grove, B. and Lockett, H. (2010) 'Mental health and employment: key opportunities to put policy into practice', www.scmh.org.uk/pdfs/mh_employment_key_opportunities.pdf

Black, C. (2008) *Working for a healthier tomorrow*, London: The Stationery Office.

Bolton, D. (2007) *What is mental disorder? An essay in philosophy, science and values*, Oxford: Oxford University Press.

Bowers, L. (1998) *The social nature of mental illness*, London: Routledge.

Boyce, M., Lockett, H. and Bacon, J. (2009) 'Mental health practitioners' role in supporting people to maintain their jobs', *Mental Health Today*, October, pp 22-6.

CMH (Centre for Mental Health) (2007) *Mental health at work: Developing the business case*, London: CMH.

Coe, L. (2009) 'Exploring attitudes of the general public to stress, depression and help seeking', *Journal of Public Mental Health*, vol 8, no 1, pp 21-31.

Depression Alliance (2008) *The inside story: The impact of depression on daily life*, London: Depression Alliance.

Deverill, C. and King, M. (2009) 'Common mental disorders', in S. McManus, H. Meltzer, T. Brugha, P. Bebbington and R. Jenkins (eds) *Adult psychiatric morbidity in England, 2007: Results of a household survey*, Leeds: The NHS Information Centre for Health and Social Care.

DH (Department of Health) (2010) *Realising the benefits. IAPT at full roll out*, http://bit.ly/pYDPYC

DWP (Department for Work and Pensions) (2008) *No one written off: Reforming welfare to reward responsibility*, Norwich: The Stationery Office.

DWP (2009) *Realising ambitions: Better employment support for people with a mental health condition*, Norwich: The Stationery Office.

Foresight Mental Capital and Wellbeing Project (2008) *Final project report – executive summary*, London: Government Office for Science.

Fournier, J.C., De Rubeis, R.J., Hollon, S.D., Dimidjian, S., Amsterdam, J.D., Shelton, R.C. and Fawcett, J. (2010) 'Antidepressant drug effects and depression severity: a patient-level meta-analysis', *Journal of the American Medical Association*, vol 303, no 1, pp 47-53.

Friedli, L., Oliver, C., Tidyman, M. and Ward, G. (2007) *Mental health improvement: Evidence based messages to promote mental wellbeing*, Edinburgh: NHS Health Scotland.

Goss, F. and Goss, D. (1998) 'The Disability Discrimination Act and SMEs: the future of the threshold', *Journal of Small Business and Enterprise Development*, vol 5, no 3, pp 270-80.

Gray, P. (1999) *Mental health in the workplace. Tackling the effects of stress*, London: Mental Health Foundation.

Haslam, C., Atkinson, S., Brown, S.S. and Haslam, R.A. (2005) 'Anxiety and depression in the workplace: effects on the individual and organisation (a focus group investigation)', *Journal of Affective Disorders*, no 88, pp 209-15.

Health, Work and Wellbeing Directorate (2008) *Improving health and work: Changing lives*, Norwich: The Stationery Office.

Health, Work and Wellbeing Directorate (2009) *Working our way to better mental health: A framework for action*, Norwich: The Stationery Office.

Henderson, M., Glozier, N. and Holland Elliott, K. (2005) 'Long term sickness absence', *British Medical Journal*, vol 330, pp 802-3.

HM Government (2009a) *New horizons: A shared vision for mental health*, London: Department of Health, www.dh.gov.uk/prod_consum_ dh/groups/dh_digitalassets/@dh/@en/documents/digitalasset/ dh_109708.pdf

HM Government (2009b) *Work, recovery and inclusion. Employment support for people in contact with secondary mental health services*, London: National Mental Health Development Unit, http://nmhdu.org.uk/ silo/files/work-recovery-and-inclusion.pdf

Hill, D., Lucy, D., Tyers, C. and James, L. (2007) *What works at work? Review of evidence assessing the effectiveness of workplace interventions to prevent and manage common health problems*, Leeds: Corporate Document Services.

Honey, A. (2002) 'The impact of mental illness on employment: consumers' perspectives', *Work*, vol 20, no 3, pp 267-76.

Horwitz, A. (2007) 'Distinguishing distress from disorder as psychological outcomes of stressful social arrangements', *Health*, vol 11, no 3, pp 271-89.

HSE (Health and Safety Executive) (2010) 'Self-reported work-related illness and workplace injuries in 2008/09: results from the Labour Force Survey', Caerphilly: Health and Safety Executive, www.hse. gov.uk/statistics/lfs/lfs0809.pdf

Irvine, A. (2008) *Managing mental health and employment*, DWP Research Report 537, London: Department for Work and Pensions.

Irvine, A. (2011) 'Something to declare? The disclosure of common mental health problems at work', *Disability & Society*, vol 26, no 2, pp 179-92.

Karp, D. (1996) *Speaking of sadness*, Oxford: Oxford University Press.

Kirsh, B. (2000) 'Organizational culture, climate and person-environment fit: relationships with employment outcomes for mental health consumers', *Work*, vol 14, pp 109-22.

Law, M., Cooper, B., Strong, S., Stewart, D., Rigby, P. and Letts, L. (1996) 'The person-environment-occupation model: A transactive approach to occupational performance', *Canadian Journal of Occupational Therapy*, vol 63, no 1, pp 9-23.

Lelliott, P., Tulloch, S., Boardman, J., Harvey, S., Henderson, M. and Knapp, M. (2008) *Mental health and work*, London: Royal College of Psychiatrists.

Leach, J. (2009) 'Diverse approaches to mental health and distress', in J. Reynolds, R. Muston, T. Heller, J. Leach, M. McCormick, J. Wallcraft and M. Walsh (eds) *Mental health still matters*, Milton Keynes: Open University Press.

MRC (Medical Research Council) (2010) *Review of mental health research. Report of the Strategic Review Group*, London, MRC.

Mental Health Foundation (2008) *How to look after your mental health*, London: Mental Health Foundation, www.mentalhealth.org.uk/publications/?entryid5=63403&char=H

NICE (National Institute for Health and Clinical Excellence) (2009) *Promoting mental wellbeing through productive and healthy working conditions: Guidance for employers*, London: National Institute for Health and Clinical Excellence, www.nice.org.uk/nicemedia/live/12331/45893/45893.pdf

Payton, A.R. (2009) 'Mental health, mental illness, and psychological distress: same continuum or distinct phenomena?', *Journal of Health and Social Behaviour*, vol 50, no 2, pp 213-27.

Pittam, G., Boyce, M., Secker, J., Lockett, H. and Samele, C. (2010) 'Employment advice in primary care: a realistic evaluation', *Health and Social Care in the Community*, 24 May, pp 1-9.

Purdon, S., Stratford, N., Taylor, R., Natarajan, L., Bell, S. and Wittenburg, D. (2006) *Impacts of the Job Retention and Rehabilitation Pilot*, DWP Research Report No 342. Leeds: Corporate Document Services.

Robertson, S. (2005) *Stress and mental health in the workplace*, London: Mind.

Rolfe, H., Foreman, J. and Tylee, A. (2006) *Welfare of farewell? Mental health and stress in the workplace*, NIESR Discussion Paper 268, London: National Institute of Social and Economic Research.

Sainsbury, R., Irvine, A., Aston, J., Wilson, S., Williams, C. and Sinclair, A. (2008) *Mental health and employment*, DWP Research Report 513, London: Department for Work and Pensions.

Sanderson, K. and Andrews, G. (2006) 'Common mental disorders in the workforce: recent findings from descriptive and social epidemiology', *Canadian Journal of Psychiatry*, vol 51, no 2, pp 63-75.

Seymour, L. (2010a) 'Common mental health problems at work: applying evidence to inform practice', *Perspectives in Public Health*, vol 130, no 2, pp 59-60.

Seymour, L. (2010b) *Common mental health problems at work. What we know about successful interventions. A progress review*, London: Centre for Mental Health.

Seymour, L. and Grove, B. (2005) *Workplace interventions for people with common mental health problems*, London: British Occupational Health Research Foundation.

Shaw, L. and Polatajko, H. (2002) 'An application of the occupation competence model to organizing factors associated with return to work', *Canadian Journal of Occupational Therapy*, vol 69, pp 158-67.

Singleton, N., Bumpstead, R., O'Brien, M., Lee, A. and Meltzer, H. (2001) *Psychiatric morbidity among adults living in private households, 2000*, London: The Stationery Office.

Taylor, R. and Lewis, J. (2008) *Understanding the impact of JRRP for people with mental health conditions*, DWP Working Paper No 45, Leeds: Corporate Document Services.

Thomas, T., Secker, J. and Grove, B. (2003) *'Getting back before Christmas?' Avon & Wiltshire Mental Health Partnership Trust job retention pilot evaluation*, Final Report to the Department of Health and Department for Work and Pensions, London: Institute for Applied Health & Social Policy, King's College London.

Underwood, L., Thomas, J., Williams, T. and Thieba, A. (2007) 'The effectiveness of interventions for people with common mental health problems on employment outcomes: a systematic rapid evidence assessment', in *Research Evidence in Education Library*, London: EPPI-Centre, Social Science Research Unit, Institute of Education, University of London.

Waddell, G. and Burton, A.K. (2006) *Is work good for your health and well-being?*, London: The Stationery Office.

Waddell, G. and Burton, A.K., and Kendall, N.A.S. (2008) *Vocational rehabilitation. What works, for whom and when?*, London: The Stationery Office.

Westerhof, G. J. and Keyes, C.L.M. (2010) 'Mental illness and mental health: the two continua model across the lifespan', *Journal of Adult Development*, vol 17, no 2, pp 110-19.

Wilson, A. and Beresford, P. (2002) 'Madness, distress and postmodernity: putting the record straight', in M. Corker and T. Shakespeare (eds) *Disability/postmodernity: Embodying disability theory*, London: Continuum.

FOUR

Comparing health and employment in England and the United States

David Lain

Introduction

This chapter addresses the role played by health in later life, especially in the context of pressures on people to remain in employment through their 60s and beyond. The 2010 Comprehensive Spending Review indicated that the state pension age (SPA) is to start rising above 65 as early as 2018, reaching 66 in 2020 (HM Treasury, 2010). This means that many people in their mid–50s today will have to work longer than either anticipated or planned. In the meantime, the government is encouraging continued employment by phasing out the default retirement age of 65. As a result, with a few exceptions employers will be forbidden from retiring staff on the basis of their age by October 2011 (BIS, 2010). This represents a considerable policy shift for the UK. Age discrimination legislation was not introduced until 2006, following an EU directive, and this only gave employees the right to *request* employment past age 65 (Sargeant, 2006). The rationale given for the impending changes includes '… demographic change; the financial benefits [of working] to both the individual and the wider economy; and the health and social benefits many people gain from working later into life' (BIS, 2010, p 5).

While the financial and health benefits of working are used as a rationale for extending working life, surprisingly little is known about how health and wealth interact to influence employment past 65. This has led to an imperfect understanding of whether employment past 65 in the coming years is feasible for those in most need of earning in later life. In general, health is likely to have exerted a particularly strong influence on continued employment in the UK. Qualitative research by Vickerstaff suggests that line managers have been crucial in deciding who can continue working past normal retirement age, typically basing decisions on the perceived interests of the firm (Vickerstaff et al, 2003;Vickerstaff, 2006a, 2006b). Research on the impact of the 2006 legislation suggests it has done little to alter the domination of a 'business case approach' to allowing continued employment (Flynn, 2010).This is likely to limit opportunities to continue working for poorer workers. Those on low incomes are likely to have worse health than their better-off counterparts (see Marmot et al, 2010) and managers have, without much difficulty, been able to confine continued employment to the healthiest, most productive staff members. Furthermore, even when they have comparable health limitations, poorer people will find it harder to continue working because they are more likely to have physically demanding, manual jobs for which there is strong competition from the core-age workforce.

In the US, on the other hand, established policies to encourage older people to continue working may mitigate the influence of health on employment past 65. The upper age limit on age discrimination legislation was abolished in the mid-1980s (Neumark, 2003). Employers can dismiss staff on the basis of diminished productivity, but not legally on the basis of age (Neumark, 2003). Without a straightforward age mechanism for sifting out staff, US employers are likely to continue employing people with health limitations for longer, and therefore in larger numbers, compared with the UK. Almost all over-65s are covered by Medicare health insurance (Salganicoff et al, 2009), reducing their dependence on employment relative to younger people. At the same time, US policy denies poorer individuals with health problems realistic financial pathways out of employment. Means-tested benefits for those with low retirement incomes are difficult to access and provided at very low levels (Lain, 2011). Therefore, although poorer people with health limitations face a number of disadvantages in terms of remaining in work, their employment in the US is expected to be closer to that of wealthier individuals.

This chapter therefore compares the influence of health and wealth on employment past 65 in the US and England, the largest country of the UK. First, consideration is given to the challenge of examining the influence on health on employment in older age with particular attention to the selection of suitable health measures. Second, employment rates at different levels of health are compared *between countries*, to see whether, as expected, employment was higher in the US. Third, the chapter compares how the influence of health on employment is played out differently depending on wealth and educational level *within* countries. A key finding is that although employment is considerably higher for those with health limitations in the US, *within* the US the poorest face considerable health and education barriers to employment. This suggests that the 'financial benefits' of working following the abolition of the UK default retirement age are likely to be limited for those in most need of additional income.

Background: measuring the impact of health on employment in the UK

While research on the impact of working conditions on health can be traced back to the 19th century, it was only much more recently that studies have explored the influence of health on employment (Griffiths, 2003). In particular, a concern with early retirement from the late 1970s onwards led to a series of UK studies exploring the degree to which it could be explained by ill health rather than choice. In contrast, studies on people working past typical retirement age have been limited in number (for a discussion see Smeaton and McKay, 2003, p 5; and McNamara and Williamson, 2004, p 259). Good health, the presence of academic qualifications and financial position all appear to be key factors influencing continued employment in older age (Parries and Sommers, 1994; Haider and Loughran, 2001; Smeaton and McKay, 2003; McNamara and Williamson, 2004). However, with the exception of a study by the present author (Lain, 2011), only Smeaton and McKay (2003) have applied quantitative measures to assess the impact of health on employment past SPA for the UK. Using the British Household Panel Survey, the authors reported that 14-15% of those rating themselves as having 'excellent' health were in employment, compared with 4-5% for those in 'poor' health. A subsequent logistic regression analysis of the Family Resources Survey found that those in 'good health' were twice as likely to work as those in 'poor health'. However, education had a strong effect independent of health. Furthermore, low levels of savings reduced the likelihood of working after controlling for other factors, something also found by Lain (2011) more broadly in relation to wealth.

US research by McNamara and Williamson (2004) suggests that self-rated health measures of the kind used above are problematic when it comes to older populations. They find that the negative effect of 'poor health' on employment decreases for men between ages 60-67 and 68-80 (McNamara and Williamson, 2004, pp 269-70). The authors attribute this to the fact that people interpret 'good health' on the basis of what they think this means for their age group. For older age groups, there is therefore likely to be a disconnection between 'good health' and employability. As corroborating evidence, respondents with a functional limitation were less likely to report themselves as being in 'poor' health if they were in the older 67–80 age group (McNamara and Williamson, 2004, p 270). It is therefore possible that the importance of health on employment past 65 might be downplayed to a degree by relying on this type of self-rated measure. This dampening effect may be strongest for lower socioeconomic groups, if they base their health assessments on social networks comprising individuals in similar circumstances to themselves (see Marmot et al, 2010 for a review of health inequalities).

Early retirement studies in the UK offer few suitable alternative quantitative measures of health that can be used with the over-65s. These have often explored the degree to which ill health is given by respondents as an *explanation* for early retirement (Laczo et al, 1988). Parker (1980, p 14), for example, highlighted the importance of health factors in premature retirement. In his study, the majority of men and women leaving work five years before SPA cited ill health as the main reason (this excluded the unemployed). However, this does not take into account the health of those *remaining* in work, some of whom may be working while successfully managing a health condition. Additionally, people are likely to have a range of explanations they can draw on for being economically inactive (Vickerstaff, 2006b, p 457). People of 'working age' may emphasise health problems where they feel this is a socially acceptable explanation for their inactivity (Johnson and Falkingham, 1992). In older age, on the other hand, retirement might be the optimal explanation for inactivity irrespective of health limitations.

Broader research on the impact of health on employment has shown that economic inactivity rates attributed to disability or ill health are also likely to be influenced by economic and policy factors. Piachaud (1986), for example, using census data, found a sharp increase in disability between 1971 and 1981. Strong correlations between unemployment and rises in disability led him to conclude that while 'objective' disability probably declined over the period, '...the impact of worsening labour market conditions has been an increase in the proportion of men seeking and settling for the status of disabled' (Piachaud, 1986, p 158). During this period, a large segment of working-age men made redundant were moved on to disability benefits because they were more generous and less stigmatising than unemployment benefits.

Ironically, therefore, it may be best to use health measures that do not make specific reference to economic status or employment when measuring the impact of health on employment. A study by Faggio and Nickel (2003) shows that the proportion of working age men claiming to have an illness or disability limiting the kind of *work* they can do rose from the early 1980s to the 2000s. However, the proportions with a limiting long-standing illness (LLSI) that limits the kinds of 'things people normally do' remained fairly stable over the period. In this context, the rise in disability benefits can be explained by the fact that low-skilled jobs declined, and low-skilled workers with a LLSI found it harder to get a job and were moved on to invalidity/incapacity benefit.

Research therefore suggests that health is likely to exert an important influence on employment, but this is likely to be played out differently depending on skill level and financial position. This relationship in turn is likely to be influenced by the economic and policy context, for example the availability and types of financial pathways out of employment (Ebbinghaus, 2006). Therefore, to better understand the influences of policy on employment, the UK needs to be compared with a country with a different set of policy arrangements. In doing so, it is important to use measures of health that do not make reference to economic activity or inactivity, or that simply ask respondents to rate their health.

Country context and data

This chapter compares the US and the UK for reasons of both policy difference and data availability. From a policy perspective, long-standing US age discrimination legislation protects individuals from forced retirement, and compels employers to continue contributing to pensions held by employees working past 65 (Quadagno and Hardy, 1991, p 473).[1] This second factor addresses some of the potential disincentives to continue working for those with salary-related pensions (Meadows, 2003). As a result, therefore, employment for those with health limitations is expected to be higher in the US than the UK.

In addition, financial pathways out of work for those with low retirement incomes and poor health are limited in the US (Lain, 2011); therefore employment of the poorest groups is expected to be closer to that of the wealthiest. Poorer individuals with health problems would be limited to applying for general means-tested benefits, but these are difficult to access and provide for a very low standard of living. In the early 2000s, the period covered here, only around one tenth of over-65s living alone or in a couple received means-tested benefits, compared with around one third in the UK.[2] US state pension entitlements were slightly less modest for those on low earnings; someone on half average earnings with full contributions records would be entitled to a state pension of 29% of average earning in the US compared with 25% in the UK (Whitehouse, 2003, p 35).[3] However, this is only a partial explanation for low levels of benefit receipt. Additionally, US income assistance benefits were not provided until the individual had very low levels of capital/savings, and were withdrawn altogether at low levels of income.[4] Likewise, US housing benefits were less generous than in the UK and were rationed, with only a small fraction of those with low incomes managing to receive help after typically queuing for years (OECD, 2004a; Priemus et al, 2005). In contrast to the US, it has been suggested that UK means-tested benefits – at least for the period covered in the research reported here – provided some degree of disincentive to employment (OECD, 2006). There is some support for this assertion: median means-tested benefits for single people over 65 were £54 per week in 2002 (DWP, 2004, p 33), and these benefits would be mostly lost as a result of earning a wage of £54 or more.[5]

The analysis provided here focuses on the year 2002 to reduce the impact of wider temporal factors influencing higher rates of US employment. As in the UK, Americans had access to a state pension at 'full' replacement rate at 65 in 2002;[6] after this they had to wait longer (so employers would probably allow people to work beyond 65 irrespective of broader policy). In addition, potential labour market demand for older workers is likely to have been similar in both countries in 2002: unemployment levels were similar,[7] and research covering a slightly earlier period suggests that the industrial composition of employment was also similar (OECD, 2000, pp 89-90).

When comparing employment past 65 in the different contexts of the UK and US, it is important to remember that not *all* of the differences in employment can be attributed to the policies cited. For example, some Americans may have been under greater financial pressure to work because Medicare health insurance did not cover out-patient prescription costs, despite being near universal for over-65s (Salganicoff et al, 2009); UK prescriptions are free for those over 60. In relation to labour market demand, lower unemployment in the US in the years *leading up* to 2002 may have contributed to a higher build-up of employment past 65 in the early 2000s (Lain, 2011).

The surveys used for this analysis, the English Longitudinal Study of Ageing (ELSA) and the US Health and Retirement Study (HRS), collect comparable data on a range of health, education, income and wealth measures (Banks et al, 2006, p 2037; Lain, 2011). The surveys, which interview people from their 50s upwards alongside their partners, have sufficiently large samples of over-65s to conduct meaningful analysis (5,538 in England and 10,428 in the US).[8] Cross-sectional weights were used in order to ensure the results were representative of the populations under investigation. Although ELSA excludes Scotland, Wales and Northern Ireland, the analysis should broadly reflect the UK situation because the vast majority of Britons, more than 80%, live in England (National Statistics, n.d.).

Comparing the influence of health on employment between England and the US

To start with the first question: were people with comparable health conditions or limitations more likely to work in the US than in England? Two measures used in both surveys are examined that meet the condition of being unrelated to work or economic activity. The first asks respondents if they have ever been diagnosed with a range of health conditions. These are presented in Table 4.1, alongside the proportions with each condition working past 65. The definition of work has a high degree of consistency between countries, asking individuals if they did any paid work or self-employment currently (in the US) or in the last month (in the UK).

Table 4.1 shows that, as expected, employment levels for those with health conditions were considerably higher in the US. It also shows that health diagnoses were higher in the US. This is consistent with research by Banks et al (2006) using the same data reporting higher rates of diabetes, hypertension, strokes and cancer among white Americans aged 55-64. Analysis of biological survey data by the authors also finds significantly higher levels of diabetes and higher risks of future

Table 4.1: Percentages of those aged 65+ ever diagnosed with various conditions, and percentages of those diagnosed in employment, England and US, 2002

	A % diagnosed		B % of diagnosed employed	
	England	US	England	US
High blood pressure	44.7	57.1	5.2	14.8
Diabetes	9.4	17.7	3.9	14.1
Cancer	7.9	16.9	5.6	14.8
Lung disease	7.9	10.5	3.7	10.9
Heart problems	28.9	30.8	4.1	14.1
A stroke	9.4	10.6	3.9	8.6
Psychiatric problems	4.9	13.0	5.6	11.0
Arthritis	39.3	65.5	3.7	15.4
None	21.9	9.4	11.2	28.0
All over-65s	N/A	N/A	6.8	17.7
Base	5,529.0	10,412.0		

Note: Bases for the percentages with different diagnoses vary slightly according to the numbers answering the question.

Source: Author's analysis of the ELSA 2002, and the US HRS 2002 (RAND Version F file).

cardiovascular problems (high levels of c-reactive protein, fibrogen and cholesterol). However, it is debatable whether health differences between countries were as big as Table 4.1 suggests for all conditions listed. According to Table 4.1, arthritis affects a majority of over-65s in the US, and a minority in the UK; it appears to have little impact on employment in the US compared with the population over 65 as a whole, but dramatically reduces the likelihood of employment in the UK. This suggests that arthritis is being diagnosed or reported for individuals with less severe joint problems than in the UK. Consistent with this, previous research indicates that US clinicians can reach very different diagnostic conclusions to their British counterparts, being more likely to recommend surgery or medication when presented with identical case histories (see Fitzpatrick, 2008 for a discussion; see also Chung et al, 2010, in relation to arthritis). A greater willingness to diagnose, and therefore treat, health conditions may in part be influenced by the US system of healthcare that financially rewards clinicians for performing health procedures and investigations (see Fitzpatrick, 2008, pp 315-16). It may also reflect differences in the cultural context, for example, the cultural appropriateness of clinicians making reference to particular medical conditions (for example, psychiatric problems).

Leaving aside the issue of comparability, it is questionable whether diagnoses are the best measure for assessing health constraints on employment. For example, having had a diagnosis of cancer in the past does not *necessarily* affect your functional work ability today (Short et al, 2008). Conditions such as arthritis may have an important influence on employment because of the constraints they may place on physical movement. Indeed, for those below SPA, musculoskeletal disorders are the single biggest physical health reason for receipt of Incapacity Benefit (Black, 2008, p 43). However, degree of physical capability, whether influenced by arthritis, cancer or some other condition, may be captured by asking people if they have difficulties doing a range of different 'activities of daily living'. This is the second health measure in both surveys. It represents a more appropriate measure of health and has been used in a number of US studies (see, for example, Haider and Loughran, 2001). A range of daily activities included in both surveys is listed in Table 4.2.

The measures in Table 4.2 are subjective in the sense that people need to judge their physical capability. However, there is little reason for assuming that all else being equal Americans are more likely to cite difficulties than Britons. The proportions citing difficulties are fairly similar for the most part, the main exception being 'walking several blocks', which can be explained by different question wording used in

Table 4.2: Percentages of those aged 65+ reporting difficulties with various activities, and percentages of those reporting difficulties in employment, England and US, 2002

	A % with difficulty with various activities		B % with difficulty employed	
	England	US	England	US
Sitting for two hours	14.7	19.4	4.1	13.4
Climb several flights of stairs	47.4	51.1	3.7	13.4
Stooping/kneeling/crouching	45.9	49.7	3.8	13.6
Difficulty lifting/carrying 10lbs	34.7	26.1	2.0	8.9
Picking up coin	7.1	8.1	1.8	9.6
Reaching/extending arms up	13.5	17.7	2.6	9.9
Pushing/pulling objects	24.5	28.5	1.7	8.7
Getting up from a chair	32.6	43.0	4.0	13.1
Walking several blocks	17.8	36.1	0.7	9.2
None	30.9	25.7	11.6	26.3
All over-65s	N/A	N/A	6.8	17.7
Base	5425.0	10396.0		

Note: Bases for the percentages with different difficulties vary slightly according to the numbers answering the question.

Source: Author's analysis of the ELSA 2002, and the US HRS 2002 (RAND Version F file).

England (this activity is therefore excluded from subsequent analysis). The questions are not asked in relation to employment, so it is likely to be a fairly stable measure of health. Activities of daily living also allow us to use a gradiated measure of health. The minority citing no difficulties are likely to have very good health, while summing the number of difficulties people report gives us a measure of the degree to which their range of physical activities are constrained.

Having established a suitable cumulative health measure, Figure 4.1 shows that in both countries employment declines as the number of health limitations increases. However, at each health level employment was higher in the US than in England, as expected. For example, at four health limitations there is still a substantial gap in employment rates (around 14% in the US and 4% in the UK). The degree of difference between countries is important. It indicates that national context is a key influence on the number of people working with health limitations. Our previous discussion suggested that policy differences would be important for explaining variations in employment. However, a key test of this is whether differences in cash benefit availability mean that wealth mediates the influence of health on employment differently in each country; this is examined in the next section of this chapter.

Figure 4.1: Employment by number of health limitations

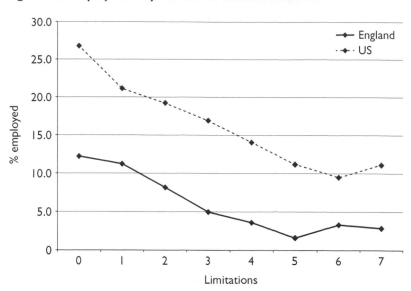

Source: Author's analysis of the ELSA 2002 and the US HRS 2002 (RAND Version F file)

The influences of health, wealth and education on employment

Although poorer people with health limitations face a number of disadvantages in terms of remaining in work, it was predicted that their employment in the US would be closer to that of wealthier individuals because of the weakness of financial pathways out of work. In order to investigate this, Figure 4.2 shows employment ratios at different levels of health – the percentage in employment in the bottom two wealth quintiles divided by the percentage in employment in the top three quintiles. These can be interpreted as the likelihood of someone with low to modest levels of wealth working relative to wealthier individuals. Wealth is presented at individual level, and relates to assets – for example, savings, investments, property and businesses (but excludes pension assets because there is no comparable data for both countries). Where a person lived with a partner their combined wealth was divided between both individuals, and adjusted to take into the account the economies of scale that come from living as a couple.[9]

In both countries, when poorer over-65s had no health limitations they worked in fairly similar numbers to their richer counterparts. Employment ratios show that the likelihood of those in the poorer category working was 79% of that of the richest in UK and 87% in

Figure 4.2: Employment ratio – bottom two wealth quintiles:top three quintiles

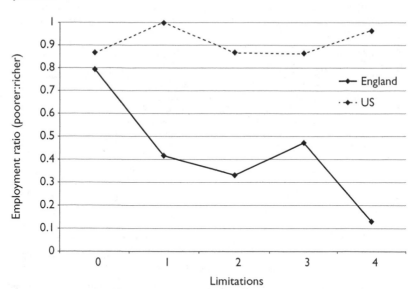

Source: Author's analysis of the ELSA 2002 and the US HRS 2002 (RAND Version F file)

the US. However, in the UK this very healthy minority of poorer individuals was the exception. The likelihood of poorer people working falls to around half that of richer individuals at one health limitation. This is as expected, given that the majority of these individuals would be entitled to means-tested benefits. In the US, where such benefits are more difficult to access and are at a lower level, the likelihood of the poorest 40% working remains much closer to that of the richer segment.

Figure 4.2 may, however, give a somewhat misleading impression of poorer people's ability to overcome health limitations and maintain financial independence by working in the US. Although poorer individuals have similar employment rates to richer individuals when they have equivalent levels of health, it is likely that the poorest have more health limitations than wealthier individuals. Likewise, it is also probable that low levels of education contribute to a lower level of employment among the poorest. Figure 4.3 shows employment ratios at different levels of health for those with low qualifications – below secondary level – relative to those with 'medium/high qualifications'. In both countries, having qualifications at secondary level or above reduces the impact of poor health on employment. With less marketable qualifications, the poorly educated may be confined to more precarious jobs at earlier ages, and once out of the labour market may find it

Figure 4.3: Employment ratio – low:medium/high education

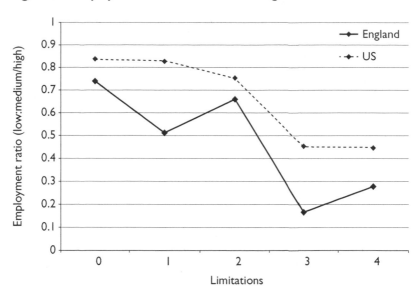

Source: Author's analysis of the ELSA 2002 and the US HRS 2002 (RAND Version F file)

difficult to return. Having qualifications may reduce the degree to which individuals' employment options are limited to physically demanding work. The influence of this factor may be reduced to a degree for the very healthy, hence the smaller difference in employment rates between educational levels for those with no health limitations. However, comparatively few over-65s have no health limitations, as was seen in Table 4.2.

Returning to Figure 4.3, it is therefore possible that the relationship between health and employment for poorer individuals is not fully captured because of inequalities in health and education. Furthermore, it is possible that the results in Figure 4.4 mask some variation between those with modest and very low retirement incomes because the bottom two wealth quintiles have been combined. Therefore a more disaggregated analysis of the influence of wealth on employment is given next, with odds ratios from logistic regression analysis that control for differences in health and education.

Employment by the poorest: constrained by education and health?

Figure 4.4 presents logistic regression odds ratios showing the relative likelihood of people over 65 working at different levels of wealth; the

Figure 4.4: Employment by wealth quintile (odds ratios controlling for age, health and educational differences)

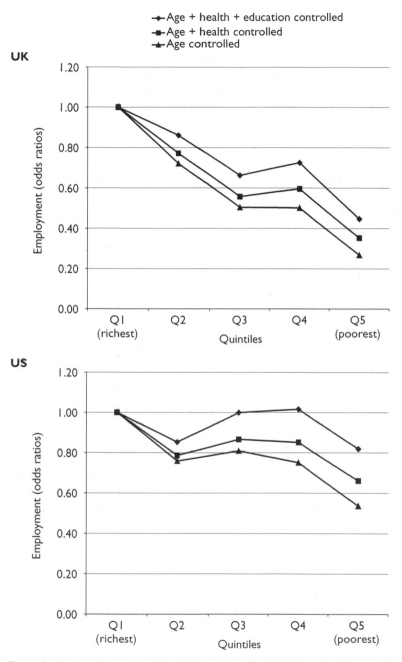

Source: Author's analysis of the ELSA 2002 and the US HRS 2002 (RAND Version F file)

richest fifth are used as the reference group against which other groups are compared.[10] The dependent variable is whether the individual aged 65-plus is employed (a value of 1) or inactive (a value of 0). The benefit of using odds ratios is that differences between wealth groups potentially influencing their employment can be controlled for. The independent 'control' variables are age in years, number of health limitations (as per Figures 4.1 and 4.2) and qualifications. The qualifications variable has three categories: 'low' (below secondary); 'medium' (secondary level to below degree); and 'high' (degree or above).[11]

Starting with England, a strong general trend of declining employment as wealth declines is evident, irrespective of the factors that are controlled for. The bottom line controls for age alone, in case poorer people's lower likelihood of employment can be explained purely because they were older; this is evidently not the case. Controlling for age, the poorest fifth had only 27% the likelihood of working of the richest (with an odds ratio of 0.27 significant at the $p<0.001$ level). Even after controlling for age, education and health, the poorest still had less than half the likelihood of working of the richest (an odds ratio of 0.45 significant at the $p<0.001$ level).

In the US, despite protection from forced retirement and greater financial need, the poorest fifth were only around half as likely to work as the richest (controlling for age; an odds ratio of 0.54 significant at the $p<0.001$ level). When differences in health between the quintile groups are controlled for, however, the difference in the likelihood of the poorest working relative to the richest falls from 46% to 34%.[12] After additionally controlling for education, the poorest are only 18% less likely to work than the richest (a difference that is significant at the $p<0.05$ level). When they have comparable levels of health and education, the poorest work in similar numbers to the richest; they *do not* have comparable health and education, however. The UK policy context appears to discourage employment past 65 *to a degree*, otherwise employment rates of poorer individuals would be closer to that of richer people after controlling for health and educational differences; however, the US example confirms that lower levels of education and health limit the ability of the poorest to work.

Conclusion

UK retirement policy is to undergo considerable change in the coming years, with people increasingly expected to work past their mid-60s. Recent announcements within the Comprehensive Spending Review 2010 indicate that the SPA is to rise faster than initially planned, from

65 to 66 between 2018 and 2020 (eventually reaching 68). This means individuals who are in their mid–50s today will have to wait longer for a state pension, and have greater financial need to work after age 65. The upper age limit of 65 on age discrimination legislation, the 'default retirement age', is also to be removed in 2011. Such a move, it is hoped, will enable people to reap financial and health benefits from working.

In this rapidly changing context, it is important to understand the factors facilitating and constraining employment. Research suggests that health, education and wealth are currently important influences on employment past typical retirement age. There is a need to improve our understanding of these influences, and this includes exploring different measures of health used. Furthermore, it is hard to assess how much influence UK policy has had on the employment of older people with health limitations due to a lack of comparative studies incorporating countries with different policy arrangements.

This chapter has therefore compared the influence of health on employment past age 65 in the US and England, the largest country of the UK. For policy reasons, the US is the ideal comparison country; age discrimination legislation covering the over-65s has a long history. Furthermore, because financial pathways out of employment are difficult to access for those with low retirement incomes, we can assess the degree to which poorer people with health conditions in the UK are 'discouraged' from working by receipt of benefits. This leads us to predict first that employment past 65 would be considerably higher in the US than England for those with comparable health limitations, and second, that despite difficulties remaining in employment, the proportion of poorest working would be closer to that of the richest in the US.

The analysis presented shows that, as expected, Americans were much more likely to work than their British counterparts with identical health limitations (measured using difficulties with activities of daily living). Furthermore, in contrast to England, when poorer Americans over 65 had comparable levels of health and education to the richest, they worked in similar numbers. However, because the poorest *did not* have comparable levels of health and education, they were much less likely to work; someone in the bottom wealth quintile was only around half as likely to work as someone in the top fifth.

This finding has important implications for UK policy. The abolition of the UK default retirement age has been justified partly on the basis of economic benefits of working to the individual. However, in the US, relatively few poorer individuals over 65 manage to maintain employment, despite the harsh financial consequences of ceasing work. As a result, despite protection from forced retirement, poverty is more prevalent in the US than the UK among older people (affecting around a sixth of over-65s in the US, compared with a tenth in the UK; Smeeding and Sandström, 2005, p 167). It is therefore imperative that extending age discrimination legislation and SPA above 65 does not lead to a reduction in financial support for the poorest, who may struggle to remain in paid employment.

Notes

[1] The law applies as long as the employer has 20 or more staff, and covers virtually all occupations (the exceptions primarily being where safety is an issue; see Macnicol, 2006, p 237).

[2] Calculated by the author using the UK Family Resources Surveys 1999-00, 2000-01, and 2001-02 (combined to increase the sample size), and the March 2001 Current Population Survey. The exact proportions were 29.8% for the UK and 10.2% for the US. This included income assistance (the UK Minimum Income Guarantee and US Supplemental Security Income), UK Council Tax Benefit, housing subsidies and benefits, and US food stamps.

[3] This is based on analysis of pension entitlements of the working-age population in the early 2000s. The State Earnings Related Pension was replaced by the State Second Pension in April 2002, which will be more generous to low earners in the long term (see Agulnik, 1999), but will not remove the need for means-tested benefits within the system.

[4] In 2002, recipients were only allowed assets of around $2,000 excluding housing to receive US Supplemental Security Income (SSA, 2003, p 2), compared with £12,000 for UK Minimum Income Guarantee (McConaghy et al, 2003, p 2).

[5] The exception to this would be £5 earnings disregards contained in the benefits (Lain, 2011).

[6] Americans could get a pension at a reduced replacement rate from 62. In the UK, women could get a pension at normal replacement rate before 65, from 60. In both countries, state pensions could be deferred or taken in full while working.

[7] Unemployment rates were 5.9% and 5.6% (for US men and women, respectively) and 5.6% and 4.4% (for UK men and women) (OECD, 2003).

[8] In the case of the HRS the Rand Version F file was used, because the data had been expertly cleaned and missing values imputed (see

St Claire et al, 2006); this was also performed for the standard ELSA data files used (ELSA, n.d).

[9] The couples income was equivilised to the individual level using the 'OECD-modified scale' (OECD, n.d), based on the premise that a couple needs 1.5 times the income of an individual to have an equivalent standard of living.

[10] Logistic regression allows us to assess the relationship, or 'effect', of one independent variable on employment, while holding still or taking into account the effects of other variables. The full regression models including age, health and education are presented in Lain (2011).

[11] This categorisation of qualification levels is based on the International Standard Classification of Education 1997 (see OECD, 2004b). Qualifications are allocated as closely as possible to ISCED 97 using information in OECD (2004b).

[12] The difference in likelihood of employment is calculated by subtracting the odds ratio for the poorest quintile from that of the richest.

Further reading

Banks, J., Marmot, M., Oldfield, Z. and Smith, J. (2006) 'Disease and disadvantage in the United States and in England', *Journal of the American Medical Association*, vol 295, no 17, pp 2037-45.

Ebbinghaus, B. (2006) *Reforming early retirement and social partnership in Europe, Japan and the USA*, Oxford: Oxford University Press.

Haider, S. and Loughran, D. (2001) *Elderly labor supply: Work or play?*, CRR Working Paper No 2001-04, Chestnut Hill, MA: Center for Retirement Research at Boston College.

Lain, D. (2011) 'Helping the poorest help themselves? Encouraging employment past 65 in England and the USA', *Journal of Social Policy*, vol 40, no 3, pp 493-512.

Smeaton, D. and McKay, S. (2003) *Working after State Pension Age: Quantitative analysis*, Department for Work and Pensions Research Report No 182, Leeds: Corporate Document Services.

References

Agulnik, P. (1999) 'The proposed state second pension', *Fiscal Studies*, vol 20, no 4, pp 409-21.

Banks, J., Marmot, M., Oldfield, Z. and Smith, J. (2006) 'Disease and disadvantage in the United States and in England', *Journal of the American Medical Association*, vol 295, no 17, pp 2037-45.

BIS (Department for Business, Innovation and Skills) (2010) *Phasing out the default retirement age: Consultation document*, London: BIS.

Black, C. (2008) *Working for a healthier tomorrow*, London: The Stationery Office.

Chung, K., Kotsis, S., Fox, D., Regan, M., Burke, F., Wilgis, E. and Kim, H. (2010) 'Differences between the United States and the United Kingdom in the treatment of rheumatoid arthritis: analyses from a hand arthroplasty trial', *Clinical Rheumatology*, vol 29, no 4, pp 363-7.

DWP (Department for Work and Pensions) (2004) *Pensioners' Income Series 2002/3*, London: DWP.

Ebbinghaus, B. (2006) *Reforming early retirement and social partnership in Europe, Japan and the USA*, Oxford: Oxford University Press.

ELSA (English Longitudinal Study of Ageing) (n.d.) *English Longitudinal Study of Ageing (ELSA): User guide for wave 1 core dataset version 2*, Documentation supplied with ELSA dataset, Essex: UK Data Archive.

Faggio, G. and Nickell, S. (2003) 'The rise in inactivity among adult men', in R. Dickens, P. Gregg and J. Wadsworth (eds) *The labour market under New Labour*, Basingstoke and New York, NY: Palgrave Macmillan, pp 40-52.

Fitzpatrick, R. (2008) 'Organising and funding health care', in G. Scambler (ed) *Sociology as applied to medicine* (6th edn), Edinburgh: Saunders, pp 313-28.

Flynn, M. (2010) 'The United Kingdom government's "business case" approach to the regulation of retirement', *Ageing and Society*, vol 30, no 3, pp 421-43.

Griffiths, A. (2003) 'Healthy work for older workers: work design and management factors', in W. Loretto, S. Vickerstaff and P. White (eds) *The future for older workers: New perspectives*, Bristol: The Policy Press, pp 212-38.

Haider, S. and Loughran, D. (2001) *Elderly labor supply: Work or play?*, CRR Working Paper No 2001-04, Chestnut Hill, MA: Center for Retirement Research at Boston College.

HM Treasury (2010) *Spending Review 2010*, Cm 7942, London: The Stationery Office.

Johnson, P. and Falkingham, J. (1992) *Ageing and economic welfare*, London: Sage Publications.

Laczo, F., Dale, A., Arber, S. and Gilbert, N. (1988) 'Early retirement in a period of high unemployment', *Journal of Social Policy*, vol 17, no 3, pp 313-33.

Lain, D. (2011) 'Helping the poorest help themselves? Encouraging employment past 65 in England and the USA', *Journal of Social Policy*, vol 40, no 3, pp 493-512.

Macnicol, J. (2006) *Age discrimination: An historical and contemporary analysis*, Cambridge: Cambridge University Press.

Marmot, M., Allen, J., Goldblatt, P., Boyce, T., McNeish, D., Grady, M. and Geddes, I. (2010) *Fair society, healthy lives: The Marmot Review, Strategic Review of Health Inequalities in England post-2010*. London: Department of Health.

McConaghy, M., Hill, C., Kane, C., Lader, D., Costigan, P. and Thornby, M. (2003) *Entitled but not claiming? Pensioners, the Minimum Income Guarantee and Pension Credit*, Department for Work and Pensions Research Report No 197, London: The Stationery Office.

McNamara, T. and Williamson, J. (2004) 'Race, gender, and the retirement decisions of people ages 60 to 80: prospects for age integration in employment', *International Journal of Aging and Human Development*, vol 59, no 3, pp 255–86.

Meadows, P. (2003) *Retirement ages in the UK: A review of the evidence*, Employment Relations Research Series No 18, London: Department for Trade and Industry.

National Statistics (n.d.) 'Census 2001', Press release, www.statistics. gov.uk/census2001/press_release_uk.asp, accessed May 2009.

Neumark, D. (2003) 'Age discrimination legislation in the United States', *Contemporary Economic Policy*, vol 21, no 3, pp 297–317.

OECD (Organisation for Economic Co-operation and Development) (n.d.) 'What are equivalence scales?', www.oecd.org/ dataoecd/61/52/35411111.pdf, accessed May 2009.

OECD (2000) 'Employment in the service economy: a reassessment', in *OECD Employment Outlook*, Paris: OECD.

OECD (2003) *Labour Force Statistics 1982-2002*, Paris: OECD.

OECD (2004a) *Benefits and wages country chapter: United States 2002*, www.oecd.org/dataoecd/4/9/34005804.pdf, accessed May 2009.

OECD (2004b) *Education at a glance 2004*, Paris: OECD.

OECD (2006) *Ageing and employment policies: United Kingdom*, Paris: OECD.

Parker, S. (1980) *Older workers and retirement*, OPCS, Social Survey Division, London, London: Her Majesty's Stationery Office.

Parries, H. and Sommers, D. (1994) 'Shunning retirement: work experiences of men in their seventies and early eighties', *Journal of Gerontology: Social Sciences*, vol 49, no 3, pp S117–24.

Piachaud, D. (1986) 'Disability, retirement and unemployment of older men', *Journal of Social Policy*, vol 15, no 2, pp 145–62.

Priemus, H., Kemp, P. and Varady, P. (2005) 'Housing vouchers in the United States, Great Britain and the Netherlands, current issues and future perspectives', *Housing Policy Debate*, vol 16, no 3 and 4, pp 575-608.

Quadagno, J. and Hardy, M. (1991) 'Regulating retirement through the Age Discrimination in Employment Act', *Research on Aging*, vol 13, no 4, pp 470-5.

Salganicoff, A., Cubanski, J., Ranji, U. and Neuman, T. (2009) 'Health coverage and expenses: impact on older women's economic well-being', *Journal of Women, Politics and Policy*, vol 30, no 2, pp 222-47.

Sargeant, M. (2006) 'The Employment Equality (Age) Regulations 2006: a legitimisation of age discrimination in employment', *Industrial Law Journal*, vol 35, no 3, pp 209-27.

Short, P., Vasey, J. and BeLue, R. (2008) 'Work disability associated with cancer survivorship and other chronic conditions', *Psycho-Oncology*, vol 17, no 1, pp 91-7.

Smeaton, D. and McKay, S. (2003) *Working after State Pension Age: Quantitative analysis*, Department for Work and Pensions Research Report No 182, Leeds: Corporate Document Services.

Smeeding, T. and Sandström, S. (2005) 'Poverty and income maintenance in old age: A cross-national view of low income older women', *Feminist Economics*, vol 11, no 2, pp 163-174 .

SSA (Social Security Administration) (2003) *SSI annual statistical report 2002*, Washington, DC: Social Security Administration.

St Clair, P., Blake, D., Bugliari, D., Chien, S., Hayden, O., Hurd, M., Ilchuk, S., Kung, F., Miu, A., Panis, C., Pantoja, P., Rastegar, A., Rohwedder, S., Roth, E. and Zissimopoulos, J. (2006) *RAND HRS data documentation, Version F*, Santa Monica, CA: RAND Center for the Study of Aging.

Vickerstaff, S. (2006a) 'Entering the retirement zone: how much choice do individuals have?', *Social Policy and Society*, vol 5, no 4, pp 507-17.

Vickerstaff, S. (2006b) 'I'd rather keep running to the end and then jump off the cliff: retirement decisions – who decides?', *Journal of Social Policy*, vol 35, no 3, pp 455-72.

Vickerstaff, S., Cox, J. and Keen, L. (2003) 'Employers and the management of retirement', *Social Policy and Administration*, vol 37, no 3, pp 271-87.

Whitehouse, E. (2003) *The value of pension entitlements: A model of nine countries*, OECD Social, Employment and Migration Working Paper No 9, Paris: OECD.

FIVE

Re-evaluating trends in the employment of disabled people in Britain

Ben Baumberg

Introduction

Experts, politicians and the public are all in agreement: there is a problem with the employment of disabled people in Britain. Over a period in which life expectancy rose, the rates of sickness benefit[1] claims increased at the same time – such that before the recent recession there were three times as many people claiming sickness benefits as unemployment benefits. This rise in sickness benefit receipt requires explanation as well as urgent intervention.

In the academic literature, there is a rough consensus over the nature of this problem, much of which stems from an influential publication in the *British Medical Journal* in 1996 (Bartley and Owen, 1996). In this paper, Mel Bartley and Charlie Owen made two observations. First, the level of disability in the British population appeared to have stayed flat over the period 1973-93. Second, the employment gap between disabled and non-disabled people increased substantially over this time. 'The problem' therefore seemed not to be one of increasing levels of disability, but rather one of changing levels of labour demand for disabled people. This analysis has not only been influential in itself, but has also been replicated and updated several times (Bartley et al, 2004; Bell and Smith, 2004; Faggio and Nickell, 2005; Berthoud, 2011).[2]

This chapter aims to show that the Bartley-Owen interpretation is partial at best, and that another explanation is possible, one that is bound up in the changing nature of work in Britain. The evidence for this is based on a superficially minor distinction about what we mean by '*disability*'. All of this previous work has looked at general measures of disability. Yet if we instead look at '*work-limiting*' disability – which reflects the *combination* of health and working conditions – we get precisely the opposite results to the established consensus. That is, the problem is *not* that employment rates among disabled people have been declining (which is what we see when we look at conventional measures of disability). Rather, *the problem is an increasing level of work-limiting disability per se* – a problem that is likely to be explained by how work has evolved over the past three decades.

This argument is developed over the course of four sections in this chapter. First, various models of disability are reviewed, with an assessment of why we should focus on work-limiting disability in particular. Second, trends in different measures of disability are analysed, both in the population as a whole and in particular subgroups. Third, trends in the employment rates of disabled people are assessed, in accordance with the different definitions outlined. Finally, the chapter considers the implications of re-evaluating the nature of the disability employment problem in the way highlighted in the analysis.

Work-limiting disability

To understand these trends, it is essential to be clear about what 'disability' actually means. The classic model of disability is that of Nagi, who separated out several related concepts (Nagi, 1965):

- pathology – the medical determination that the body is failing to work as 'normal';
- functional limitations – the inability to perform specific tasks;
- disability – the inability to perform a social role.

This is similar to the World Health Organization's more recent (2001) International Classification of Functioning, Disability and Health (Ustun et al, 2003), which makes a threefold distinction between 'body functions and structures', 'activities' and 'participation'. With such distinctions in mind, we can now consider how we might actually think of disability itself. According to the traditional 'medical model', disability is the inevitable consequence of these pathologies and functional limitations. This has successfully been challenged by the 'social model' of disability (Barnes and Mercer, 2004), where problems in performing a role are due to a disabling social context rather than the pathologies themselves. More recently, the health professions have developed the 'biopsychosocial model' (Wade and Halligan, 2004), where the disabling context is split into personal (attitudinal), social and physical aspects. These three models of disability therefore focus on different aspects of disability: the medical model emphasises health itself; the social model emphasises the expectations that society places on a person; and the biopsychosocial model emphasis individual attitudes and choices, and therefore the way in which two individuals with similar pathologies can experience different levels of disability.

Disability is, therefore, intimately linked with specific social roles – and this means that a person can be disabled for one social role (for example, 'worker') while non–disabled for another (for example, 'parent'). And crucially here, trends in the level of specific types of disability will depend on trends in the demands of the social role itself. In other words, trends in work-limiting disability depend on trends in working conditions as well as trends in pathologies.

Yet previous analyses of trends in employment among disabled people have ignored the impact of the changing nature of work, and instead equated 'disability' with 'pathology'.[3] This is not just a matter of conceptual fussiness. We have good reasons for being particularly interested in what is termed work-limiting disability (WLD), as *non*-work limiting health problems are unlikely to affect a person's employment. This is borne out by the work of Melanie Jones (Jones, 2006), who found that people with a long-standing illness but no WLD were as likely to work as those without any illnesses at all. WLD is also important over time; among people in work, those reporting a WLD are much more likely to have a health-related job loss two to three years later *even after controlling for their actual level of health*.[4] In other words, it is WLD that is important for labour force participation, and not other measures of health/disability.

This is not to say that it is pointless to examine trends in the employment of people with a given level of health. To the extent that limiting long-standing illness (LLSI) is a good approximation to 'health' in general,[5] the analyses of Bartley and Owen (and others) provide valuable evidence on whether there is an increasing employment penalty to health problems. We would also expect a substantial overlap between WLD and LLSI – after all, if people's health limits their ability to work, people will usually report that it affects their 'activities' as well (see also Manderbacka, 1998, p 323).[6] Previous research is therefore not wrong in drawing conclusions on health and employment trends, but rather does not consider that the work role has changed throughout this period. The analysis below suggests that this is of crucial importance with the final section identifying some implications for social policy.

Trends in the level of disability

This section examines trends in disability comparing the conventional measure of LLSI to WLD. To do this, the estimates of Bartley and Owen are reconstructed using the General Household Survey (GHS),[7] and analyses of WLD in the Labour Force Survey (LFS) by the author are added. This enables us to examine trends in the working-age population from 1984-2006, with two breaks in 1989 and 1997 where data could not be made comparable (see Web Appendix A and Cousins et al, 1998).[8] The overall trends in WLD and LLSI are shown in Figure 5.1. Using the conventional measure of disability (LLSI), the prevalence of disability was flat – there was a rise in the early 1990s and a fall in the late 1990s, leaving only a small rise from 14.9% to 16.1% from 1984 to 2006. This fits the results of previous research, although it is worth noting that there was an earlier rise in the 1970s (Berthoud, 2011, p 14).

In contrast, the level of WLD in 2006 is far greater (and statistically significantly greater) than in 1984 – if we piece together the three different series,[9] WLD rose from 10.1% in 1984 to 16.0% in 2006. The differences in the trends between WLD and LLSI are striking. Interestingly, the trends mirror each other, in that both were relatively stable in the 1980s and 2000s, and saw rises in the early 1990s. The

Figure 5.1: Trends in the prevalence of disability in the working-age population

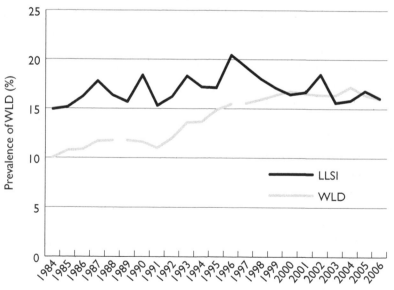

Notes: Working-age population is defined as men aged 20-64, women aged 20-59. WLD = work-limiting disability; LLSI = limiting long-standing illness.
Source: Author's analysis of weighted Labour Force Survey data; see Web Appendix A (available from www.benbaumberg.com) for details.

difference is rather in the size of the rise in the early 1990s, and the existence of a fall in LLSI – but not WLD – in the late 1990s.

While no other surveys allow us to focus so specifically on WLD, the 1991 and 2001 censuses did ask people if they had a long-term illness that 'limits your daily activities or the work you can do' – effectively a combination of LLSI and WLD. This also shows a rise over the 1990s from 7.1% in 1991 to 12.5% in 2001 among women, and from 9.4% to 14.3% among men.[10] If we accept that there was no rise in LLSI over this period, this provides yet more evidence that WLD rose sharply in the 1990s.

A potential criticism of my argument here is that there will inevitably be more people reporting a WLD if there are more people claiming sickness benefits. After all, we have suggestive evidence that non-workers are more likely to report ill health than others to (consciously or unconsciously) justify their worklessness (for example, Baker et al, 2004; Kapteyn et al, 2009), and this is likely to be particularly strong for WLD. Figure 5.2 therefore shows trends in reported WLD by economic status, excluding both the temporarily sick and long-term sick. This shows a substantial rise in WLD among the working population (the

Figure 5.2: Trends in work-limiting disability by economic status, 1984-2006

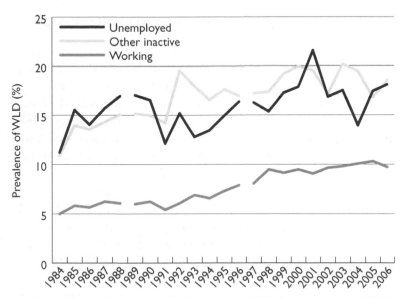

Notes: Working-age population is defined as men aged 20-64 and women aged 20-59.
Source: Author's analysis of weighted LFS data; see Web Appendix A (available from www.benbaumberg.com) for details.

rate nearly doubles to 10%), as well as rises among other inactive people in the 1980s and among unemployed people in the 1990s.

Another possible reason for rising levels of WLD is that there has been a decline in labour market demand for certain groups, making increasing numbers of health problems seem 'work-limiting' (compare Faggio and Nickell, 2005, pp 3-4). If this were the case, we would expect to see levels of WLD increasing most in those groups that have seen the biggest decline in labour demand, that is, the low-skilled. However, the relative increase in WLD among those with a degree and those with no qualifications is virtually identical, with WLD doubling in both cases.[11]

In conclusion, this section has demonstrated that disability as measured by LLSI has not risen over the period 1984-2006. At the same time, there has been a sharp rise in WLD. This rise in WLD is not because there are more sickness benefit claimants justifying their claims in 2006 than in 1984; even if we exclude these people and look only at workers, there was a near doubling of WLD over this period. The rise can also be seen in people with a degree, rather than being restricted to those with no qualifications whose labour demand has declined in recent decades. Some policy implications of this analysis are discussed in the final section of the chapter. The next section focuses on whether the falling employment rates among disabled people can still be observed if we focus on WLD rather than LLSI.

Trends in the employment rate of disabled people

The current consensus is that the employment rate of disabled people declined in the 1980s and 1990s. However, this is based on disability as measured by LLSI, which – as we have already seen – shows a markedly different trend to WLD. If we are instead concerned with disability as measured by WLD, do we still see a declining employment rate? To begin with, we can ignore non-disabled people and just focus on the employment rate among disabled people. For men, there is a striking difference between the two definitions of disability: there was an 8% *fall* during the period 1984-2006 in the employment level of men with a LLSI, but a 3% *rise* in the employment level of men with a WLD. For women, the difference is less pronounced: there was a rise in the employment level of both definitions of disabled women, although the rise was slightly higher for WLD than LLSI (8.6% versus 5.5%). However, employment rates are affected by the economic cycle and the secular rise in female employment rates – so it is perhaps clearer to look at the *employment gap* between disabled and non-disabled people using the two different definitions of disability.

Looking at the employment gap for men in Figure 5.3, we can again confirm the conventional view that there has been a rising employment gap for LLSI, from 26% to 36% over the period. Yet if we look at WLD, we see a starkly different picture: there has been no overall rise in the gap, which is 43-44% at both ends of the period.

Figure 5.3: Trends in the employment gap between disabled and non-disabled men: comparing different definitions of disability (WLD and LLSI)

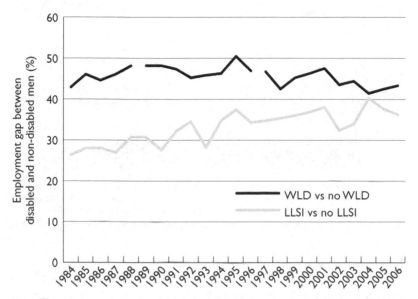

Notes: The employment gap is calculated as the employment rate among non-disabled men, minus the employment rate in disabled men. LLSI = limiting long-standing illness, based on General Household Survey (GHS) data. WLD = work-limiting disability, based on LFS data.
Source: Author's calculations based on the working-age population (men aged 20-64).

Turning to the equivalent figures for women, the estimated disabled employment gap is shown in Figure 5.4, against the background of generally rising employment. Here we can see once more the rising employment gap when we define disability as an LLSI (from 18% to 27%), but a general picture of stability when we define disability as a WLD (the gap rising only slightly from 31% to 34%).

As a final aside, it has repeatedly been noted that the decline in the employment rates of disabled people has been much greater in those with low levels of education (Bartley and Owen, 1996; Bell and Smith, 2004; Faggio and Nickell, 2005). Following the pattern of this entire chapter, the results using a WLD definition of disability are entirely

Figure 5.4: Trends in the employment gap between disabled and non-disabled women

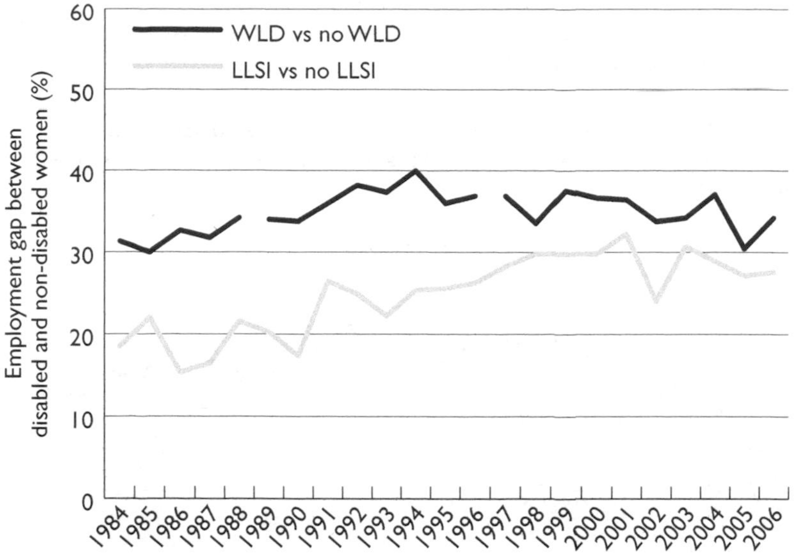

Notes: The employment gap is calculated as the employment rate among non-disabled women, minus the employment rate in disabled women. LLSI = limiting long-standing illness, based on GHS data. WLD = work-limiting disability, based on LFS data
Source: Author's calculations based on the working-age population (women aged 20-59).

different: there is no change whatsoever in the disabled employment gap for those with no qualifications.

Overview and implications

This chapter has presented the argument that the conventional view of trends in the employment rates of disabled people is partial at best. The conventional view is that the disabled employment gap – the difference in employment rates between disabled people and non-disabled people – has increased from the early 1980s to the present day (Bartley et al, 2004; Bell and Smith, 2004; Faggio and Nickell, 2005; Berthoud, 2011). In contrast, the analysis provided here shows that the disabled employment gap has barely changed for either men or women from 1984-2006. The reason for such different conclusions is that the trends are highly sensitive to how we define 'disability'. If we define disability as activity limitations, the conventional view is correct. Yet, when disability is defined as *work* limitations, the picture changes entirely. Not only is there no increase in the disabled employment gap, but we also see a rise in WLD over the 1980s and 1990s.

The difference between 'work-limiting' and conventional measures of disability is the focus on work, and an obvious explanation for any divergence between the measures is therefore based on the work role itself. Put simply, it could be *that changes in the nature of work have made a constant level of ill health more disabling at work, compared with 30 years ago.* This may seem surprising in an economy where tough manual labour has been steadily replaced by service sector work – yet there are signs that other changes in the labour market have been less benign. For example, Francis Green has shown that 'job strain' – a combination of low control over work, combined with high required effort – increased from less than 10% in 1992 to around 20% in 2006 (Green, 2009). Moreover, many – although not all – other psychosocial job stressors show similar rises over the 1990s, with data generally unavailable before this (Green, 2006; White, 2009).

The best way of dealing with a problem is not necessarily the reverse of its cause. Similarly, even if working conditions are shown to be part of the explanation for rising sickness benefit receipt, this does not necessarily mean that the best policies are focused on working conditions. In fact, we already have evidence about the effectiveness of workplace interventions in helping people with health problems to continue working (Franche et al, 2005; Chapter Six, this volume). As a result, working conditions and employer-focused interventions

Figure 5.5: Trends in job strain in Britain 1992-2006

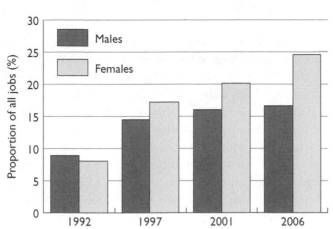

Note: 'Job strain' is where jobs have high quantitative demands (that is, compulsory work effort) and low control over the job.
Source: Green (2008)

are part of the Fit for Work agenda (Black, 2008; Chandola, 2010) – although current discussions often fail to link sickness benefits to quality of work, and entirely ignore the macro-level interventions and public sector reform that could change the nature of British jobs (see Chapters Ten and Twelve).

But the potential impact of the evidence in this chapter is less about 'what works', and more about 'what happened' – our understanding of the causes of the rise in sickness benefit receipt (see also Chapter Nine). Yet a focus on 'what happened' is no less important for policy than 'what works'. Politics is not a technocratic exercise in applying empirical findings, but a place where different narratives clash (among many other sources, see Lakoff, 2002).

Currently, the narrative is that sickness benefits cannot reflect 'real' limitations in fitness for work, given that the number of claimants has risen, while work has become less physically demanding and the population has become healthier (compare Piggott and Grover, 2009 on 'scroungerphobia'). A genuine rise in WLD is a challenge to this narrative. If confirmed, this lends support to another story, where people with health problems are excluded from the labour market by jobs that have become ever more difficult for them. This explanation is rooted in factors outside of the control of the individual, and therefore suggests they are more 'deserving' than they are currently seen – and therefore, more entitled to public support (van Oorschot, 2000).

All of this presumes that there has been a real rise in WLD caused by deteriorating working conditions – but this is not the only valid interpretation of the results in this chapter. To varying degrees, a number of other interpretations are also possible:

• Ill health could have genuinely increased. Yet although it is possible for mortality to decline while morbidity rises (Waidmann et al, 1995, p 270; PMSU, 2005, p 35), it just does not seem plausible that ill health rose on this scale.[12] Population-wide measures of specific physical and mental conditions show a mixture of declines, small rises or inconsistent trends (Wadsworth et al, 2003; McManus et al, 2009), while LLSI more generally shows no lasting increase.

• The rise of the 'work stress' phenomenon (see Chapter Nine) could have made people more likely to report a WLD. But it is important to bear in mind that people are actually much less likely today than in the early 1990s to say their work causes health problems – the rise of work stress has been counterbalanced by a feeling that work is less bad for *physical* health.[13] Perceptions of work stress may therefore play a role, but this does not mean that we now see work as necessarily more health-damaging than in the past.

- If labour demand declines, people with health problems may be pushed to the back of the 'queue for jobs' (Beatty et al, 2000) and become more likely to report a WLD, even though neither their health nor the nature of work has changed. Rising levels of WLD would therefore be a result of declining labour demand – which is already seen as a major contributor to rising sickness benefits (Beatty and Fothergill, 2005; Houston and Lindsay, 2010; Berthoud, 2011).[14]
- Rising sickness benefits are also thought to be due to changing incentives and eligibility in the benefits system, as set out in an authoritative review of US and UK research by Duncan McVicar (2008). Given that nearly all of those claiming sickness benefits report a WLD, this will have contributed to the rise in WLD – although it cannot explain the rising levels of WLD among workers.
- Similarly, different individuals have different attitudes that will influence whether they see their health problem as work-limiting, as made clear by the biopsychosocial approach. Such perceptions of WLD are often cited by politicians as a determinant of high sickness benefit levels, such as the then Secretary of State for Work and Pensions Peter Hain in 2007 arguing that: 'There are many people sitting at home in the belief that they are unemployable.... But this is just not the case.'[15] This is a difficult topic to provide robust evidence on, though, and we have little data on trends in people's attitudes to fitness for work (as separate from their *actual* fitness for work).

Conclusion

In short, this chapter on its own provides an insufficient basis to conclude that working conditions have played a major role in the rise in sickness benefits receipt in Britain. Instead, it suggests only the *possibility* that working conditions have played a role – but this is a possibility that has not previously been considered. This is not to say that working conditions have been ignored in the literature on sickness absence, work disability and return to work – clearly working conditions are known to play a major role (for example, Franche et al, 2005), and it has been suggested that trends in working conditions may explain trends in work-related stress (for example, Stansfeld et al, 2008). The point is rather that the contribution of working conditions to rising levels of sickness benefit receipt as never been formally studied, and is therefore omitted from reviews that seek to explain it (for example, McVicar, 2008). In ongoing research, I am responding to this gap by systematically reviewing data on trends in job strain and investigating in more detail how far this contributes to rising sickness benefit receipt,[16] but further research by the wider research community is also required to test the alternate explanations above.

The contribution of this chapter has been to challenge the existing narrative on disability and employment, and to suggest that deteriorating working conditions *may* have played a larger role than is currently being contemplated. It is, however, the task of future research to investigate how far working conditions did *actually* play such a role, and to ultimately determine whether our understanding of rising levels of sickness benefits receipt must be replaced by a new narrative. If working conditions are confirmed as a major factor, this suggests that policy should not only help individuals to better manage their health in work, but also consider the quality of work per se.

Notes

[1] Throughout this chapter, I follow the DWP in using the term 'sickness benefits' to refer to the benefits that are paid to people because their health limits their ability to work – namely Invalidity Benefit, Incapacity Benefit, Severe Disablement Allowance and now Employment and Support Allowance.

[2] Other analyses have noted an upturn in the employment rate of disabled people more recently (Black, 2008; Smith, 2008, p 1).

[3] For example, the work of Bartley and Owen looks at 'limiting long-standing illness', for which people with a long-standing illness were asked if their illness/disability 'limits your activities in any way'. Within Nagi's terminology, we might even question whether this is a measure of 'disability' at all rather than a measure of 'functional limitations' (although in Bartley and Owen (1996) – unlike several later authors – the term 'disability' is avoided).

[4] Author's calculations using the Whitehall II survey; see Web Appendix B for details, available from www.benbaumberg.com.

[5] LLSI is obviously only a crude approximation of this – particularly given that even activity limitations seem to be affected by societal and medical changes (Freedman et al, 2004).

[6] This is not universally true, however. In separate qualitative work within the same wider project, I found that some people with mental health problems would say that their ability to work was affected,

but that their ability to do 'activities' like sport and housework was unaffected.

[7] See Web Appendix A, available from www.benbaumberg.com.

[8] From comparisons of the results, it seems likely that some of these adjustments were not made in previous analyses of LFS data (Bell and Smith, 2004; Faggio and Nickell, 2005). Web Appendix A is available from www.benbaumberg.com.

[9] The single series is created by chaining the first value of the new series to the last value of the previous series. This assumes that trends in all the versions of the LFS WLD questions would have been identical, and that there were no changes during the discontinuities in 1988-99 and 1996-97.

[10] Estimates for the working-age population and excluding those in communal establishments. The census question explicitly asks people to 'include problems which are due to old age'.

[11] The absolute percentage point increase is nevertheless much greater in those with no qualifications, with the increases being 6% (5% to 11%) among those with degrees compared to 15% (15% to 30%) among those with no qualifications. It is for this reason that some researchers have argued that the rise in WLD is primarily among those with no qualifications (Bell and Smith, 2004, p 16; Faggio and Nickell, 2005, p 17).

[12] There was a slight decline in self-reported general health from 1984-96, but this returned to almost the original level in the period 1996-2006 (in similar fashion to LLSI). Furthermore, self-reported health will partly reflect WLD; for example, 20% of respondents to the 1984/95 Health and Lifestyles Survey cited 'work/being busy' as the most important factor in deciding how to report their own level of health.

[13] See www.hse.gov.uk/statistics/history/illhealth.htm, accessed 30 January 2011.

[14] It should be noted that WLD almost doubled among workers, and there were similar rises in the levels of WLD among both the highly-educated and the low-skilled. Nevertheless, it is plausible that labour demand plays some role.

[15] www.dwp.gov.uk/mediacentre/pressreleases/2007/nov/drc055-191107.asp, accessed 10 April 2008.

[16] For future updates on this research, see www.benbaumberg.com

Further reading

Beatty, C. et al (2000) 'A theory of employment, unemployment and sickness', *Regional Studies*, vol 34, no 7, pp 617-30.

Bell, B. and Smith, J. (2004) *Health, disability insurance and labour force participation*, Bank of England Working Paper No 218, www. bankofengland.co.uk/publications/workingpapers/wp218.pdf

Berthoud, R. (2011) *Trends in the employment of disabled people in Britain*, ISER Working Paper No 2011-03, Colchester: Institute of Social and Economic Research, University of Essex, www.iser.essex.ac.uk/publications/working-papers/iser/2011-03.

Green, F. (2006). *Demanding work: The paradox of job quality in an affluent economy*, Princeton, NJ: Princeton University Press.

Stansfeld, S.A. (2008) 'Work-related distress in the 1990s – a real increase in ill health?', *Journal of Public Mental Health*, vol 7, no 1, pp 25-31.

References

Baker, M. et al (2004) 'What do self-reported, objective, measures of health measure?', *Journal of Human Resources*, vol 39, no 4, pp 1067-93.

Barnes, C. and Mercer, G. (2004) *Disability policy: Applying the social model*, Leeds: The Disability Press.

Bartley, M. and Owen, C. (1996) 'Relation between socioeconomic status, employment, and health during economic change, 1973-93', *British Medical Journal*, vol 313, no 7055, pp 445-9.

Bartley, M. et al (2004) 'Employment status, employment conditions, and limiting illness: prospective evidence from the British household panel survey 1991-2001', *Journal of Epidemiology and Community Health*, vol 58, no 6, pp 501-6.

Beatty, C. and Fothergill, S. (2005) 'The diversion from "unemployment" to "sickness" across British regions and districts', *Regional Studies*, vol 39, no 7, pp 837-54.

Beatty, C. et al (2000) 'A theory of employment, unemployment and sickness', *Regional Studies*, vol 34, no 7, pp 617-30.

Bell, B. and Smith, J. (2004) *Health, disability insurance and labour force participation*, Bank of England Working Paper No 218, www. bankofengland.co.uk/publications/workingpapers/wp218.pdf

Berthoud, R. (2011) *Trends in the employment of disabled people in Britain*, ISER Working Paper No 2011-03, Colchester: Institute of Social and Economic Research, University of Essex, www.iser.essex.ac.uk/publications/working-papers/iser/2011-03.

Black, C. (2008). *Working for a healthier tomorrow: Dame Carol Black's review of the health of Britain's working age population*, London: The Stationery Office, www.workingforhealth.gov.uk/documents/working-for-a-healthier-tomorrow-tagged.pdf.

Chandola,T. (2010) *Stress at work:A report prepared for the British Academy*, London: British Academy Policy Centre, www.britac.ac.uk/policy/Stress-at-Work.cfm, accessed 13 February 2011.

Cousins, C. et al (1998) 'Disability data from the Labour Force Survey: comparing 1997-8 with the past', *Labour Market Trends*, vol 106, no 6, pp 321-36.

Faggio, G. and Nickell, S. (2005) *Inactivity among prime age men in the UK*, CEP Discussion Paper No 673, London: Centre for Economic Performance, http://eprints.lse.ac.uk/19912/1/Inactivity_Among_Prime_Age_Men_in_the_UK.pdf, accessed 28 August 2008.

Franche, R.-L. et al (2005) 'Workplace-based return-to-work interventions: a systematic review of the quantitative literature', *Journal of Occupational Rehabilitation*, vol 15, no 4, pp 607-31.

Freedman,V.A. et al (2004) 'Resolving inconsistencies in trends in old-age disability: report from a technical working group', *Demography*, vol 41, no 3, pp 417-41.

Green, F. (2006) *Demanding work:The paradox of job quality in an affluent economy*, Princeton, NJ: Princeton University Press.

Green, F. (2008) 'Work effort and worker well-being in the age of affluence', in R. Burke and C. Cooper (eds) *The long work hours culture: Causes, consequences and choices*, Bingley: Emerald.

Green, F. (2009) 'Job quality in Britain', Praxis 1, London: UK Commission for Employment and Skills, www.ukces.org.uk/upload/pdf/A5%20Job%20Quality%20in%20Britain%20v6.pdf, accessed 20 May 2010.

Houston, D. and Lindsay, C. (2010) 'Fit for work? Health, employability and challenges for the UK welfare reform agenda', *Policy Studies*, vol 31, no 2, pp 133-42.

Jones, M.K. (2006) 'Is there employment discrimination against the disabled?', *Economics Letters*, vol 92, no 1, pp 32-7.

Kapteyn,A. et al (2009) *Work disability, work, and justification bias in Europe and the US*, NBER Working Paper 15245, Cambridge, MA: National Bureau of Economic Research, http://www.nber.org/papers/w15245.

Lakoff, G. (2002) *Moral politics: How liberals and conservatives think*, Chicago, IL: University of Chicago Press.

Manderbacka, K. (1998) 'How do respondents understand survey questions on ill-health?', *European Journal of Public Health*, vol 8, no 4, pp 319-24.

McManus, S. et al (2009) *Adult psychiatric morbidity in England, 2007: Results of a household survey*, Leeds: NHS Information Centre for Health and Social Care.

McVicar, D. (2008) 'Why have UK disability benefit rolls grown so much?', *Journal of Economic Surveys*, vol 22, no 1, pp 114-39.

Nagi, S. (1965) 'Some conceptual issues in disability and rehabilitation', in M. Sussman (ed) *Sociology and Rehabilitation*, Washington, DC: American Sociological Association, pp 100-13.

Piggott, L. and Grover, C. (2009) 'Retrenching Incapacity Benefit: Employment Support Allowance and paid work', *Social Policy and Society*, vol 8, no 2, pp 159-70.

PMSU (Prime Minister's Strategy Unit) (2005) *Improving the life chances of disabled people: Final report*, London: Prime Minister's Strategy Unit with DWP, DH, DfES and ODPM, www.cabinetoffice.gov.uk/strategy/work_areas/disability.

Smith, D. (2008) 'Self-reported disability status, onset and employment', Paper presented at Work, Pensions and Labour Economics Study Group (WPEG) Conference 2008, http://wpeg.group.shef.ac.uk/papers2008/30Smith.pdf

Stansfeld, S.A. et al (2008) 'Work-related distress in the 1990s – a real increase in ill health?', *Journal of Public Mental Health*, vol 7, no 1, pp 25-31.

Ustun, T. et al (2003) 'The International Classification of Functioning, Disability and Health: a new tool for understanding disability and health', *Disability and Rehabilitation*, vol 25, no 11-12, pp 565-71.

van Oorschot, W. (2000) 'Who should get what, and why? On deservingness criteria and the conditionality of solidarity among the public', *Policy & Politics*, vol 28, no 1, pp 33-48.

Wade, D.T. and Halligan, P.W. (2004) 'Do biomedical models of illness make for good healthcare systems?', *British Medical Journal*, vol 7479, no 329, pp 1398-401.

Wadsworth, M. et al (2003) 'Health', in E. Ferri, J. Bynner and M. Wadsworth (eds) *Changing Britain, changing lives: Three generations at the turn of the century*, London: Institute of Education, University of London.

Waidmann, T. et al (1995) 'The illusion of failure: trends in the self-reported health of the US elderly', *The Milbank Quarterly*, vol 73, no 2, pp 253-87.

White, M. (2009) *Work orientations of older employees: Change over the 90s and into the 00s*, PSI Discussion Paper (New Series) 2, London: Policy Studies Institute.

SIX

The current state of vocational rehabilitation services

Joanne Ross

Introduction

Vocational rehabilitation (VR) is an umbrella term used to describe the wide range of processes and interventions that enable people with a health condition, injury or disability to enter, return to, or remain in work. As such, the current state of VR services is critical to the wellbeing-at-work agenda and the expected need, with an ageing population, for an even greater emphasis on enabling people with health conditions to remain in employment. This chapter examines VR interventions and the contexts in which services are delivered. Contemporary approaches to VR are discussed, including traditional condition-focused and newer occupation-focused perspectives. The discussions place a particular emphasis on how contextual factors influence practice within this field. The chapter goes on to explore how advancements in VR services have been hampered by significant challenges, not least terminological inconsistencies, shifting socio-political agendas and a traditionally reductionist approach to interventions. It then touches on the impact of historical trends on the sustained development of these types of services, together with tensions posed by factors such as a lack of professional regulation within the sector. Finally, the chapter explores the shift in focus towards early intervention and the likely impact of planned welfare reforms.

A lack of shared understanding: evidence, terminology and frameworks

Within healthcare, the ability to demonstrate the effectiveness of a particular intervention has long been highly prized. Within VR, there is the added requirement to make a business case that demonstrates the cost-effectiveness of the intervention (Joss, 2002). However, there remains a lack of consensus as to what VR means, or what it entails.

This lack of clarity has negatively affected researchers' ability to generate the substantive evidence needed to drive practice forwards in a consistent manner. This problem is coupled with the difficulties inherent in evaluating complex healthcare interventions of this kind (Campbell et al, 2000).

As a result, the literature fails to reflect an accurate understanding of the multidimensional nature of the role of return-to-work facilitators and the VR process (Shaw and Polatajko, 2002). For many years, useful descriptive accounts of well-established programmes designed to assist people into, and back to, work have been published within the international literature (Floyd, 1996; Pratt and Jacobs, 1997; O'Halloran, 2002; Koch and Rumrill, 2003; Curtis, 2003). There remains, however, a dearth of robust, large-scale comparative studies on which to build the evidence base. This section further examines some central ways in which terminological confusion and the absence of a unifying framework have imposed barriers that continue to hamper the development of a shared understanding and practice.

'Vocational rehabilitation' is widely recognised as an unwieldy term that is somewhat dated, often poorly understood and frequently unpopular with disability groups. International attempts to find a more suitable descriptor have led to a plethora of terms being applied to elements of similar interventions. References can be found to work rehabilitation, industrial rehabilitation, occupational rehabilitation, return-to-work interventions, work injury prevention, vocational practice, disability management and work practice (Matheson et al, 1985; Innes, 1995; Pratt and Jacobs, 1997; Isernhagen, 2000; Lyth, 2001; Gibson and Strong, 2003; Strong et al, 2003).

These terminological discrepancies are frequently determined by factors such as the source of the funding stream for intervention or the particular stage of recovery a person is at. Some interventions are confined to groups with a particular health condition or disability, to the exclusion of others (Williams and Westmorland, 2002; McCluskey et al, 2005). Similar anomalies are apparent when examining what VR actually entails. It is variously described as a process, an array of services, a service model, a form of intervention and a type of programme (Wehman and Kreutzer, 1990; Perron and Mckay, 1997; Dean et al, 1999; Danner et al, 2000; Kumar, 2000; Allaire et al, 2003; Frank and Thurgood, 2006). The UK has tended to hold a wider understanding of VR than that found in most other countries, yet there remains a clear need for a common terminology to facilitate understanding and opportunities for meaningful applied research (College of Occupational Therapists, 2003; Barnes and Holmes, 2007; Ross, 2007).

Exploration of the professional literature also reveals that VR has different meanings to different groups within the various sectors in which it is delivered. For example, a qualitative research project by Irving et al (2004) presented findings from the differing perspectives of employers, insurers, solicitors and providers. Within the confines of their study, the category of providers was described in somewhat avaricious terms as having

> ... an interest in providing a commercially viable service which they can 'sell' to employers, insurers and solicitors. Providers working with large companies/organisations justify their existence by reducing the levels of absence and getting staff back to work sooner using VR processes and interventions. (Irving et al, 2004, p 1)

This commercially biased description fails to accurately reflect the acknowledged contribution made by practitioners, such as health professionals, within the sector.

The lack of a unifying theoretical framework poses further challenges. A 20-year review of the literature on work outcomes revealed that studies in this field were set within a fragmented and disorganised knowledge base that lacked any theoretical underpinnings (Shaw and Polatajko, 2002). There has been a failure to consistently apply recent and relevant theory to work and VR practice. As a result, there continues to be 'A major need for well-documented evidence about frameworks, models, or protocols that will provide evidence of successful vocational rehabilitation strategies' (Kumar, 2000, p 278).

The former UK government attempted to provide direction and leadership within the sector, through a planned programme intended to present an overview of current work, define the scope of VR and develop a framework for effective intervention. The resultant policy, outlined in *Building capacity for work: A UK framework for vocational rehabilitation* (DWP, 2004), did indeed produce definitions, but failed to put forward the long-awaited, unifying framework. Primarily targeted at those already in employment, the framework document was not instrumental in creating widespread change and the intended reforms failed to materialise (Curtis, 2007; Black, 2008). The inconclusive evidence base for VR played a significant role in this lack of progress.

Approaches to vocational rehabilitation

The elusiveness of a unifying theoretical framework or model for VR means that it is dominated by traditionalist approaches. VR services delivered in healthcare settings continue to adopt a condition-focused perspective. This has, in many ways, served to fragment the knowledge base still further, since medical diagnosis alone is a poor indicator of an individual's likelihood or ability to return to work. Making this point, Dyck and Jongbloed (2000) 'concluded that the availability of social resources within the work environment can have a greater impact on employment status than the diagnosis or severity of a particular disease alone.

Condition-focused approaches seek primarily to gain an understanding of a disease process, impairment or disability. They include conceptualisations about the nature, aetiology, anticipated course and management of the condition, as well as associated implications for the individual's present and future functioning. Perceived capacity for work is shaped by these understandings. Modern-day ailments most commonly resulting in sickness absence include musculoskeletal and mild-to-moderate mental health conditions (Waddell and Burton, 2006). The origins and nature of these conditions means that an underlying organic pathology is rarely identified. They continue, therefore, to pose a challenge to established diagnostic reasoning.

Application of biopsychosocial models has produced alternative explanations drawn from psychological theories. They have increasingly linked these widespread conditions with some form of faulty thinking or disease misconception (Verbeek, 2006). Contemporary suggestions as to their cause have included cognitive factors, health beliefs or illness perceptions, and ruminating or catastrophising about pain (Petrie et al, 1996; Sullivan et al, 1998; Daniels et al, 2004). Others have argued that they stem from some sort of illness behaviour (Mechanic, 1995). An increasing emphasis on individual responsibility and freedom of choice has led some to suggest that sufferers may, in some way, be choosing illness (Galvin, 2002) or intentionally producing symptoms to seek secondary gains, such as support and care (Egmond, 2005). The presence of symptoms not fully explained by disease has led to these conditions variously being labelled as a form of illness deception (Halligan et al, 2003) or a 'nonphysical socio-political phenomenon' (Ireland, 1998, p 63).

These views collectively highlight the shortcomings within traditional medical and psychological models. Since subjective health conditions account for three quarters of self-reported, non-fatal, work-related illnesses, seeking alternative ways of understanding is essential. The need for a fresh approach, able to respond to the changing trends in the nature and prevalence of work-related health and disability, has been recognised (Waddell and Burton, 2006).

The discussion so far is not to suggest that the nature of the health condition is unimportant, but rather that this is just one of many factors that may affect a successful return to work. All too often, too little attention is paid to understanding the wider impact of the condition on the individual concerned and to 'bridge the divide between health and occupation' (Alsop, 2004, p 525).

The *illness experience* affects how a person adapts to the change in circumstances brought about by their condition (Ross, 2008). Individuals develop their own unique understanding and way of responding to a health situation. There are multiple internal and external factors that may influence a given individual's particular response. Personal experiences, pre-existing health beliefs and the views of others, combined with learned abilities to deal with adversity, will differ. As a result, the process of adjustment involved in coming to terms with a chronic health condition, and the limitations it imposes, is a very individual process. The illness experience has the potential to be a significant barrier to return to work.

A disability or chronic health condition emerging at some point in the lifespan inevitably has a disruptive impact on the person. It may affect not only their functional motor, cognitive and sensory skills, but also their occupational identity, through an associated inability to participate in valued, meaningful everyday activities or 'occupations'. It is important to recognise than any given individual carries out a unique blend of activities and occupations that make up their daily existence (Kielhofner, 2008). The diversity of these occupations is infinite, ranging from leisure activities like snowboarding, fishing or reading; through routine personal self-care and hygiene activities such as showering or bathing; to paid work activities with a particular set of demands and expectations attached to them. Together, this unique blend of activities makes up a person's *occupational identity*, which extends beyond their work life. It includes the roles, routines and balance of the particular occupations the person performs on a day-to-day basis.

Occupational identity is underpinned by the value and meanings that an individual attaches to these daily occupations within the wider social context in which they occur. It may be surmised that their worker identity forms an element of their wider occupational identity. *Worker identity* captures the person's perception of themselves, as a worker or potential worker, together with the fears, values and meanings they attach to work (Ross, 2008). This identity is not static as suggested by some (Neff, 1976; Kielhofner, 2008), but is subject to dynamic transitions. It shifts and evolves, suggesting that it may diminish or be strengthened over time. Any effective welfare-to-work programme must recognise the need, at an individual level, to build a worker identity where one is absent. If not recognised and addressed in a timely manner, levels of motivation, feelings of fear, uncertainty or sometimes ambivalence, may all have a negative effect on the outcome of a VR intervention.

In the discussion mentioned earlier, attention is drawn to important intrinsic characteristics of the person that are all too frequently overlooked in attempts to move people into, or back to, work. However, an occupation-focused perspective of VR must extend beyond merely this understanding of the person. It calls for congruence between the characteristics of the individual within their wider everyday life, the qualities and features of their work, and the demands of the workplace. This occupational profile extends to include the goodness of fit between the worker, their work and key factors within the workplace environment (Shaw and Polatajko, 2002).

Vocational rehabilitation: contextual dimensions of practice

Historical trends towards investment, and disinvestment, in VR programmes are apparent. In the past, the greatest enabler of these programmes was the advent of a major war, the purpose of VR being to support the return of injured and disabled soldiers back to as normal a civilian life as was possible. Large workshops with simulated work activities were used to physically recondition soldiers in preparation for life and work on the outside. Their success resulted in expansion into civilian hospitals (Hanson and Walker, 1992).

Within the wider population, the focus of rehabilitation shifted during the 1970s and 80s. There was an increased emphasis on the development of skills for independent community-based living, as asylums and residential homes for the disabled were closed. There was little expectation of work, with a minority of the more able-bodied being offered places in sheltered workshops that were segregated according to the nature of the disability (Ross, 2007).

VR has traditionally been afforded higher priority during times of economic strength. Unsurprisingly, therefore, the buoyant state of the economy has added significant momentum to service growth in recent years. Coupled with a renewed interest in work, health and disability, modern-day VR has been driven forwards by a wealth of social policy that, directly and indirectly, has shaped how, where and what, services are being delivered. The highlighted links between poverty, health inequalities, social exclusion and long-term unemployment have served to add further impetus to the expansion of services designed to help those with a health condition or disability back into the workplace. The recognition of the stigma and discrimination faced by people with disabilities and health conditions, in particular those with mental health conditions (Repper and Perkins, 2003), has led to the creation of new models of support and increased opportunities for individuals to enter paid work.

Within the confines of current competitive recruitment processes, employment law and welfare benefit restrictions, however, too little opportunity for innovation in practice remains. The application of techniques such as job carving, for example, would help to ensure greater labour market participation for those with a chronic, but currently stable, health condition or disability. Creating a job based on an identified workplace need, but designed specifically with an individual in mind, will enable the person's particular functional strengths and limitations to be most effectively matched. This kind of approach would require a significant paradigm shift away from current employment practices.

Objective measures of health, such as life expectancy and morbidity, have improved over the past quarter of a century. Despite this, the number of people claiming health-related disability benefits has trebled to well over 2.5 million (DWP, 2002 and Chapters Seven and Eight of this volume). As many as 27,000 people leave employment permanently each year after becoming ill or sustaining an injury at work (TUC, 2002) and the UK reportedly has the second highest number of workers suffering from long-term sickness in the European Community (*People Management*, 2004). Setting aside the problems inherent in the measurement and definition of health (see Chapters Four and Five), published figures paint a bleak picture of the current state of the health of the UK's working-age population. When coupled with increasing life expectancy, the implications for individuals, industry and our society as a whole are immense.

The determination of health status based solely on subjective self-assessments needs to be treated with a degree of caution, since individuals' perceptions of the state of their health are likely to fluctuate over time (Atkinson et al, 2007). Notwithstanding these uncertainties, as many as **two million** people report suffering from an illness which they believed was caused, or made worse, by current or past work, with more than a quarter of these being reported in the space of a year (HSE, 2007). Improved opportunities for earlier VR, as recommended by the Health and Safety Commission (HSC, 2000), are of particular importance as ways to increase workforce productivity are sought.

The culture of long work hours (TUC, 2007), increased job intensity and discord between co-workers means that the incidence of subjective health complaints, such as work-related stress, has continued to rise (HSC, 2006; see also Chapter Nine of this volume). The current downsizing of the public sector workforce, and the associated threat to job security, will add to the stress experienced by this sizeable workforce. To counteract these strains, investment in coordinated and effective workplace health and wellbeing programmes is essential.

The insurance sector has been a growth market for VR services. With one of the largest insurance sectors in the world, UK companies operate within a very competitive market. For example, income protection insurance, taken out by companies that want to protect themselves against the financial loss resulting from an employee's illness, injury or death, saw payouts in the region of £1 billion in 2004 (Wright et al, 2005). Income protection and employers' compulsory liability insurers and those covering healthcare, such as personal medical and motor insurance products, may all potentially benefit from what rehabilitation can offer (Waddell and Burton, 2004), with VR having a central role to play in this powerful economic marketplace.

The potential for harm to occur in the workplace means that an element of the expressed concern for workers' health and safety comes from rising compensation claims, under, for example, compulsory employers' liability insurance schemes. This trend has affected the insurance sector and employers alike. Large compensation payouts are highly visible in the media, amid ongoing fears of the development of the 'compensation culture' found in America. An influential report (Better Regulation Task Force, 2004) suggested that the fear of litigation leads to over-cautiousness among employers, as well as being a drain on time and money. A need was identified for a more efficient system of redress when people's rights are infringed, without the accompanying blame culture that seeks out the person 'at fault' when things go wrong. One of the recommendations of the task force was the investigation of mechanisms enabling earlier access to rehabilitation. The recent government review, *Common sense common safety* (Young, 2010), recommends tighter controls in the sector but misses the opportunity to spell out how VR can contribute to better outcomes.

The need to reform employers' liability insurance is widely recognised, the argument being that key changes, such as a shift away from a culture of lengthy personal injury claims seeking large financial settlements towards the potential benefits of VR and better occupational health services, would help more people return to work earlier and more effectively (Association of British Insurers, 2005). The 1999 Rehabilitation Code of Practice, updated in 2007, provides an approved framework for injury claims, promoting rehabilitation early on in the compensation process, thereby supporting the best and quickest possible medical, social and psychological recovery (Association of Personal Injury Lawyers, 2004). The code is not, however, mandatory and as such its adoption has not been universal. Calls for the 'provision of enough financial support to increase the number of rehabilitation specialists' (Association of British Insurers, 2005, p 1) have also largely gone unheeded.

The different contexts in which vocational rehabilitation occurs

In the UK at present VR occurs in a number of different institutional settings, which has implications for the nature of interventions. In this section we consider the key findings from a doctoral study that explored the re-emerging role of occupational therapy within VR in the UK (Ross, 2008). Qualitative case-study methodology was used to allow a deeper understanding to be gained of practice within, and across, different settings identified as centres of excellence in VR. A combination of interviews, observations and document analysis provided insights into VR, with a particular focus on the occupational therapy contribution to the team and the wider service. Using a multiple case-study design, four organisational case studies were undertaken sequentially. Each built on, consolidated and challenged the themes that emerged from within each setting. Cross-case data analysis and synthesis was organised according to Carney's Ladder of Analytical Abstraction (1990 in Miles and Huberman, 1994, p 92), enabling the analysis to be undertaken at organisational, operational and conceptual levels, guided by the theoretical propositions and research questions. Key findings from the case studies were grouped into themes, illustrating how the person, their work and the workplace may be understood within a VR intervention. The different settings for VR will be discussed in turn.

Case study one: the insurance company

The global presence of this multinational organisation allowed it to learn the benefits of VR through international experience. Drawing on expertise from countries such as Australia and New Zealand, the company's UK VR service dated back to 2001. Since that time, it had placed an increasing emphasis on maximising the effectiveness of interventions and publicising and promoting the value and benefits of this approach. Success in this endeavour had resulted in a doubling in the size of the rehabilitation team, to around 40 staff, since its inception.

This VR service was funded through income protection insurance. Within the UK, the organisation provided this type of cover to over two million people. The product was primarily purchased by larger companies that wished to protect themselves, and in some instances their employees' income, against financial loss arising from injury, illness or death, regardless of cause. Common practice holds that income protection insurers only become financially liable as statutory sick pay ends, six months after an insured absence has begun. This insurance company, however, provided an additional service to key customers, in the form of a pre-claim early intervention service. By facilitating an earlier return to work the likelihood of a long-term absence was reduced.

The primary purpose of the VR was to facilitate a timely and successful return to work with selected individuals. Health professionals from a variety of backgrounds, mainly occupational therapy, were generically called vocational rehabilitation consultants. Using a case-management model, practitioners addressed primarily long-term absence and its associated costs. Support was provided to employees and employers during the development of a return-to-work plan and through the transition back to work, together with advice about disability-related issues where necessary.

Participation in a VR programme was voluntary, with periodic file reviews helping to identify potentially suitable candidates. VR could be offered at any point after a claim had been approved. In addition to case management and early intervention, the service operated an assessment unit for functional capacity and ergonomic assessments. Independent external consultants, usually with an occupational therapy or physiotherapy qualification, were commissioned to undertake these activities.

The theme 'facilitation of the return to work' described the steps involved in the VR intervention, with the intended outcome of the intervention being a return to employment with the existing employer.

A further theme, 'understanding the worker', highlighted the ways in which condition-focused knowledge, for example functional performance abilities and the impact of the health condition on function, was synthesised with occupational knowledge, such as occupational identity, introduced earlier in the chapter. Familiarisation with 'the work/job' involved seeking an understanding of the structure and function of the work itself. Gathering this information allowed the practitioner to make a formulation as to the likely fit between the two domains of the worker and their work, together with any potential barriers or risks involved in a return to work. The final theme in this case study, 'the workplace', recognised the need for the practitioner to gain knowledge of the work environment and also to have sufficient business acumen to understand the employer's perspective.

Case study two: the occupational health team

This service was sited within the public acute healthcare sector, in an NHS hospital that employed around 4,500 staff. Its purpose was to provide in-house occupational health services to its staff, of whom approximately 70% were women. In contrast to the large rehabilitation team within the insurance company, this small occupational health team reflected the familiar structure found within traditional healthcare environments. It comprised a service manager and administrative staff, occupational health nurses, an occupational therapist, sessional doctors, a psychologist and a holistic therapist. A part-time physiotherapist was soon to join the team.

Emergent themes from this case study included 'the workplace and the perspective of the employer' and 'getting both sides of the story'. These built on the theme of 'the workplace' identified in the first case study. The pivotal role of the employer was highlighted, as was the need for the practitioner to actively seek to gain their collaboration with the VR process. Being based at the worksite allowed the occupational therapist in this role to gain an expert knowledge of the workplace, to form effective working relationships with staff, and to assess the nature of the actual work tasks from an insider perspective.

The theme 'the work/job: an understanding of everybody's role' encompassed the need to analyse and understand the functional requirements of the job, in order to ascertain how duties could be modified to accommodate a particular injury or disability. These assessments, in turn, informed the development of the rehabilitation plan and 'facilitating the return to work'. For a successful outcome to be achieved, the practitioner needed to be recognised as fair and impartial by all parties involved in the return-to-work plan. The final theme, understanding 'the worker as a person', reinforced the need for a holistic understanding beyond merely the work role or the health condition.

Case study three: the condition management programme

In this setting, a team of over 50 occupational therapists, nurses, physiotherapists and other allied health professionals, most of whom were expert clinicians, were generically employed as condition management practitioners. The service had been running for five years, and formed part of the first wave of pilot sites within the wider Department for Work and Pensions' Pathways to Work scheme (Barnes and Hudson, 2006). The service, starting with just a handful of staff, had seen rapid expansion across the region and its success meant that a national roll-out of the condition management programmes was being implemented at the time of the fieldwork.

The service was delivered as a partnership between the local NHS and Jobcentre Plus. Individuals using the service were unemployed 'customers' moving on to long-term health-related benefits (formerly known as Incapacity Benefit [IB]). They were required to attend a series of mandatory work-focused interviews with a personal adviser at Jobcentre Plus. One of the options available was attendance on a condition management programme. These programmes, underpinned by a biopsychosocial model, used a cognitive-behavioural approach as the basis for the intervention (Newman et al, 2004; Waddell and Aylward, 2005).

Themes emerging from this case study added further to an understanding of the person. In common with previous case studies, it was necessary to 'overcome mistrust' at the outset of the intervention. The setting illustrated the difficult 'route to recovery', or journey back to work, for this group. Thus there was a need to 'build a worker identity' before work-seeking activities could begin. 'Work and the workplace' were understood in much broader terms than, for example, in case study two. In this setting, training, voluntary work and work schemes were all recognised as stepping-stones towards paid employment, which was the stated aim of the Pathways to Work programme as a whole. In contrast to the second case study, there was a visible gap at the critical interface between the practitioner and the workplace, with employer engagement being undertaken by others as a separate process.

This shortcoming failed to recognise the ongoing needs of those with a long-term health condition in securing and retaining work, as well as the vital role of the employer in delivering a successful outcome. The value of local labour market knowledge was highlighted, as was the shortage of good-quality employment. Short-term contract work and care work for the minimum wage often held little appeal, illustrating the mismatch between employer requirements and individuals' worker identity and aspirations.

Case study four: a private rehabilitation company

The final case study setting was an independent rehabilitation case management company providing national coverage. In common with case study one, funding for this medical and vocational rehabilitation service came from within the insurance sector. The customer base was made up of a number of insurance companies, each commissioning a rehabilitation case management service for an insured individual who was the victim of either physical or psychological injury.

Established three-and-a-half years previously, the company had expanded rapidly year on year. Nearly 60 practitioners, mainly with an occupational therapy or physiotherapy background, were employed as generic rehabilitation case managers. The majority had trained outside the UK and described being able to make a difference to individuals' lives by recommending, coordinating and overseeing the delivery of a variety of interventions directed towards their recovery. The theme 'pathway to recovery for work' conceptualised this process differently from that encountered in case study three, with clear distinctions being made between return to work with an existing employer and seeking a new job. The use of this traditional Australian model drew attention to how professional training and practitioners' prior experience influenced service design and delivery.

A degree of data saturation was discovered during this case study. Additional themes that emerged, beyond those identified previously, included 'commercial awareness and business acumen' and 'the case manager role'. Practitioners worked to targets, billed for their time and were frequently required to defend and justify their recommendations to others. The need for confidently assertive communication skills, beyond a level generally required from allied health professionals working in traditional healthcare settings, was apparent.

In summary, the themes identified within each of the four case studies provided a rich, descriptive account of the core components of vocational rehabilitation. Further cross-case analysis enabled the development of conceptual definitions of both the process and the intervention involved in this form of rehabilitation. This, in turn, has added to existing understandings in this complex field of practice.

Sustainability: workforce dimensions and the state of the economy

The increased demand for VR in recent years has highlighted the need for practitioners with the right skill set to deliver these interventions. For example, concerns were raised that just 400 occupational therapists in the UK undertook VR as a primary part of their role (Wright et al, 2005). It is likely that there had been some expansion of this number in the intervening years, but this small number of rehabilitation practitioners must be viewed in the context of a situation with over two-and-a-half million people on long-term health-related benefits. Of these, just under a third, roughly 800,000 people, were predicted likely to need specialist disability support to be able to work (British Society of Rehabilitation Medicine, 2003). Many more are away from, or struggling to remain in, work because of their health condition or disability.

Pointing to the need for educational reform, the view that 'as work awareness is required in all NHS professions it needs to be part of the undergraduate training of all NHS staff. Those who need a greater input are undergraduate doctors, occupational therapists and physiotherapists' (British Society of Rehabilitation Medicine, 2000, p 63), remains a challenge to achieve (Ross, 2006).

Concerns about capacity within the sector are heightened by the unease surrounding competency. While rehabilitation professionals such as occupational therapists are state-regulated, with the accompanying accountability and standards of practice, there are no such boundaries or safeguards with respect to VR. Concerns raised by member organisations such as the Vocational Rehabilitation Association and others have highlighted the growing number of provider companies and practitioners in the field with no professional qualifications whatsoever. It is perfectly legal for anyone to call themselves a VR practitioner. Jobs in the sector are seldom advertised as profession-specific, as highlighted in the earlier case studies. Titles such as vocational, or employment, consultant or vocational case manager are commonplace. The emergence of new hybrid interdisciplinary models, such as workplace disability management (Shrey and Hursh, 1999; Harder and Scott, 2005), work injury management and disability prevention (Isernhagen, 2000) serve to illustrate a growing miscellany of approaches that compounds this problem.

This unsatisfactory situation has prompted calls for the accreditation of education and training in VR. These views are supported by those in the insurance sector who have called for 'a transparent accreditation system for rehabilitation qualifications' (Association of British Insurers, 2005, p 1). This would, it is argued, produce competent practitioners who are fit for practice, while ensuring that required standards are met. Attempts in recent years to introduce greater standardisation have seen the introduction of common international terms, professional standards and codes of practice (Vocational Rehabilitation Association, 2006, 2007; United Kingdom Rehabilitation Council, 2009; Escorpizo et al, 2010). While these initiatives are to be welcomed, the absence of any national requirement for accreditation means that safeguarding arrangements remain unsatisfactory.

History reflects how disinvestment in VR services is linked with economic recession. In the UK recession in the 1980s, for example, most forms of rehabilitation for work were dropped from the agenda. At the time, political disinterest, coupled with a weak economy and the decline of certain industries, meant that work was in short supply, especially for large numbers of people with disabilities regarded as being incapable of work. VR was, to all intents and purposes, largely a thing of the past. This decline in the provision of rehabilitation by occupational therapists was in contrast to the situation in a number of other western countries where the contribution of occupational therapists within the workplace was well documented and has remained well established (Mountain et al, 2001). The recent surge of demand in the UK has drawn heavily on the skills of therapists trained overseas to meet this need.

The impact of economic conditions is further illustrated in the changing fortunes of one of the previous government's flagship welfare to work initiatives. The Green Paper *Pathways to Work: Helping people into employment* (DWP, 2002) was aimed at the 700,000 people who moved from paid work on to long-term IB each year. Seven pilot schemes, introduced in late 2003, were underpinned by the notion that, with the right help and support, significant numbers of people may be prevented from coming on to IB, or alternatively, helped off it and back into work. The condition management programme in one such pilot site was described earlier in the chapter. The pilot was delivered in a time of economic prosperity with the associated increase in the availability of work, particularly in the service sectors. Evaluations of the Pathways to Work pilot outcomes were positive, as they increased the numbers leaving IB and returning to employment by 9% (Waddell and Aylward, 2005; DWP, 2007). As a result of this success, pilot status ended in spring 2006 and a phased national roll-out of the programme was undertaken. The tide has, however, turned and a recent report by the Public Accounts Committee strongly criticised the Pathways programme for relying on an over-optimistic impression of what could be achieved. Unlike the pilots, the majority of the new services were commissioned from private providers who seriously underperformed against contracts and achieved lower success rates than Jobcentre Plus. In 2008-09, £94 million (38% of Pathways expenditure) was spent on employment support that did not in fact enable people to enter employment. By March 2010, the scheme had cost an estimated £760 million, with the numbers on IB dropping by just 125,000 between 2005 and 2009, including those helped back to work by Jobcentre Plus (Public Accounts Committee, 2010).

It is clear that the current recession, coupled with the alternative ideological stance of the incumbent government, is likely to produce a shift towards state disinvestment in VR services in the coming years. The impact on other sectors is, as yet, less clear-cut.

Looking to the future: benefit entitlement, early intervention and prevention

Recent reforms of the benefit system, including new medical assessment procedures, have set a threshold whereby nearly 40% of new claimants for long-term health-related benefits are deemed capable of work. This tightening of entitlement is intended to reduce the 2.6 million claimants in this category. With fewer people eligible, there is likely to be a knock-on increase in the numbers claiming Jobseeker's Allowance (JSA). Although it is too soon for a definitive evaluation of the impact of these and further planned reforms, anecdotal evidence suggests that general practitioners have seen a concurrent rise in the numbers of patients on JSA seeking sickness certification. These individuals consider themselves too ill to be in work, even when the state has deemed them fit. No provision has been made for VR services to support this group in their recovery for work.

It is interesting to reflect on this change, especially when a rise in the number of people counted as unemployed rather than as incapable of work has often been a politically unpalatable reality in the past. This shift in stance contrasts visibly with the introduction of long-term health-related benefits in the 1980s, which had the effect of masking the true scale of job losses and unemployment levels at that time (see Chapter Seven).

The 2008 Black review made a number of recommendations intended to improve the health of the working-age population. These saw the fit note replace the sick note for those signed off work by their GPs, as well as several pilot sites testing Fit for Work Services. Further impetus was added by the Boorman review (DH, 2009) into the state of the health and wellbeing of the NHS workforce. The importance of early intervention to prevent job loss has been a core theme of the recommendations. While it is too early to speculate on the outcome of these initiatives, active engagement and collaboration between the employee, health professionals, GPs, occupational health services, employers and their representatives, and others, are all crucial to their success. Modern VR services hold the key to bringing these diverse stakeholders together through negotiated, outcome-focused return-to-work plans. There is, however, no 'one size fits all' solution. To be successful, these arrangements must be personalised to the needs of the individual and their unique occupational identity, taking into account the work duties they perform and the wider context of their workplace environment. This review of the current state of VR services in the UK, while covering some examples of good practice, does not allow for any complacency over the readiness of VR services to cope with the current levels of work-limiting ill health or the extra demands of an ageing population who will be expected to work for longer.

Further reading

Frank, A.O. and Thurgood, J. (2006) 'Vocational rehabilitation in the UK: opportunities for health-care professionals', *International Journal of Therapy and Rehabilitation,* vol 13, no 3, pp 126-34.

Harder H.G. and Scott L.R. (2005) *Comprehensive disability management,* Edinburgh: Churchill Livingstone.

Holmes J. (2007) *Vocational rehabilitation,* Oxford : Blackwell Publishing.

Ross, J. (2007) *Occupational therapy and vocational rehabilitation,* Chichester: Wiley.

Whiteford, G. and Wright-St Clair, V. (2005) *Occupation and practice in context,* Sydney: Livingstone Churchill.

References

Allaire, S.H., Li, W. and LaValley, M.P. (2003) 'Reduction of job loss in persons with rheumatic diseases receiving vocational rehabilitation: a randomized controlled trial', *Arthritis & Rheumatism,* vol 48, no 11, pp 3212-8.

Alsop, A. (2004) 'Work matters', Editorial, *British Journal of Occupational Therapy,* vol 67, no 12, p 525.

Association of British Insurers (2005) *Care and compensation*, London, www.abi.org.uk/Publications/ABI_Publications_Care_and_Compensation_f67.aspx

Association of Personal Injury Lawyers (2004) *Best practice guide on rehabilitation*, Nottingham: Association of Personal Injury Lawyers, www.apil.com

Atkinson, A., Finney, A. and McKay, S. (2007) *Health, disability, caring and employment: Longitudinal analysis*, DWP Research Report no 461, Leeds: Corporate Document Services.

Barnes, T. and Holmes, J. (2007) *Occupational therapy in vocational rehabilitation:A brief guide to current practice in the UK*, London: Executive Committee of the College of Occupational Therapists Specialist Section: Work.

Barnes, H. and Hudson, M. (2006) *Pathways to Work: Qualitative research on the condition management programme*, DWP Research Report 346, Department for Work and Pensions, Leeds. Corporate Document Services.

Better Regulation Task Force (2004) *Better routes to redress*, London: Cabinet Office Publications and Publicity Team.

Black, C. (2008) *Working for a healthier tomorrow*, London: The Stationery Office.

British Society of Rehabilitation Medicine (2000) *Vocational rehabilitation: The way forward*, Working Party Report, London: British Society of Rehabilitation Medicine.

British Society of Rehabilitation Medicine (2003) *Vocational rehabilitation: The way forward* (2nd edn), Report of a working party, London: British Society of Rehabilitation Medicine.

Campbell, M., Fitzpatrick, R., Haines, A., Kinmonth, A.L., Sandercock, P., Spegelhalter, D. and Tyrer, P. (2000) 'Framework for design and evaluation of complex interventions to improve health', *British Medical Journal*, vol 321, pp 694-96.

College of Occupational Therapists (2003) *Research and development strategic vision and action plan for occupational therapy in work practice and productivity*, London: College of Occupational Therapists.

Curtis, J. (2003) 'Employment and disability in the United Kingdom: an outline of recent legislative and policy changes', *Work*, vol 20, no 1, pp 45-51.

Curtis, J. (2007) 'Summary of recent and current government developments in vocational rehabilitation', *RehabReview*, March, http://rehabwindow.net/RecentNewsletters.aspx, accessed 28 April 2007.

Daniels, K., Jones, D. and Perryman, S. (2004) *Cognitive factors' influence on the expression and reporting of work-related stress*, HSE Research Report RR170. London: Health and Safety Executive.

Danner, R., Halonen, P., Juntunen, M. and Javikallio, J. (2000) 'Questionnaire test-retest reliability: outcome measure of a vocational rehabilitation programme', *International Journal of Rehabilitation Research*, vol 23, pp 245-52.

Dean, D.H., Dolan, R.C. and Schmidt, R.M. (1999) 'Evaluating the vocational rehabilitation program using longitudinal data. Evidence for a quasi-experimental research design', *Evaluation Review*, vol 23, no 2, pp 162-89.

DH (Department of Health) (2009) *NHS health and well-being*, Final Report, London: The Stationery Office.

DWP (Department for Work and Pensions) (2002) *Pathways to Work: Helping people into employment,* London: The Stationery Office.

DWP (2004) *Building capacity for work: A UK framework for vocational rehabilitation,* London: The Stationery Office.

Dyck, I. and Jongbloed, L. (2000) 'Women with multiple sclerosis and employment issues: a focus of social and institutional environments', *Canadian Journal of Occupational Therapy*, vol 67, no 5, pp 337-46.

Egmond, J. (2005) 'Beyond secondary gain', *American Journal of Psychoanalysis*, vol 65, no 2, pp 167-77.

Escorpizo, R., Finger, M.E., Glässel, A. and Cieza, A. (2010) 'An international expert survey on functioning in vocational rehabilitation using the International Classification of Functioning, Disability and Health', *Journal of Occupational Rehabilitation*, E-publication ahead of print, available at www.ncbi.nlm.nih.gov/pubmed/21152958, accessed 23 January 2011.

Floyd, M. (ed) (1996) *Vocational rehabilitation and Europe*, London: Jessica Kingsley.

Frank, A.O. and Thurgood, J. (2006) 'Vocational rehabilitation in the UK: opportunities for health-care professionals', *International Journal of Therapy and Rehabilitation*, vol 13, no 3, pp 126-34.

Freud, D. (2007) *Reducing dependency, increasing opportunity: Options for the future of welfare to work*, Independent report to the Department of Work and Pensions Leeds: Corporate Document Services.

Galvin, R. (2002) 'Disturbing notions of chronic illness and individual responsibility: towards a genealogy of morals', *Health*, vol 6, no 2, pp 107-37.

Gibson, L. and Strong, J. (2003) 'A conceptual framework of functional capacity evaluation for occupational therapy in work rehabilitation', *Australian Occupational Therapy Journal*, vol 50, pp 64-71.

Halligan, P., Bass, C. and Oakley, D. (eds) (2003) *Malingering and illness deception*, Oxford: Oxford University Press.

Hanson, C.S. and Walker, K.F. (1992) 'The history of work in physical dysfunction', *American Journal of Occupational Therapy*, vol 46, no 1, pp 56-62.

Harder, H.G. and Scott, L.R. (2005) *Comprehensive disability management*, Edinburgh: Churchill Livingstone.

HSC (Health and Safety Commission) (2000) 'Revitalising health and safety strategy', London: The Stationery Office.

HSC (2006) 'The strategy in action: report to ministers on the second year of the HSC strategy', www.hse.gov.uk/aboutus/hsc/strategyyear2.pdf, accessed 13 November 2006.

HSE (Health and Safety Executive) (2007) *Self-reported work-related illness and workplace injuries in 2005-2006*, Results from the Labour Force Survey, Caerphilly: HSE Books.

Innes, E. (1995) 'Workplace-based occupational rehabilitation in New South Wales', *Australia Work*, vol 5, pp 147-52.

Irving, A., Chang, D. and Sparham, I. (2004) *Developing a framework for vocational rehabilitation: Qualitative research*, DWP Report No 224, Leeds: Corporate Document Services.

Ireland, D.C.R. (1998) 'Australian repetition strain injury phenomenon', *Clinical Orthopaedics & Related Research*, vol 351, pp 63-73.

Isernhagen, D.D. (2000) 'A model system: integrated work injury prevention and disability management', *Work*, vol 15, no 2, pp 87-94.

Joss, M. (2002) 'Occupational therapy and rehabilitation for work', *British Journal of Occupational Therapy*, vol 65, no 3, pp 141-8.

Kielhofner, G. (2008) *Model of human occupation. Theory and application* (4th edn), Baltimore, MD: Lippincott Williams & Wilkins.

Koch, L.C. and Rumrill, P.D. Jr. (2003) 'New directions in vocational rehabilitation: challenges and opportunities for researchers, practitioners, and consumers', *Work*, vol 21, no 1, pp 1-3.

Kumar, S. (2000) *Multidisciplinary approach to rehabilitation*, Boston, MA: Butterworth Heinemann.

Lyth, J.R. (2001) 'Disability management and functional capacity evaluations: a dynamic resource', *Work*, vol 16, no 1, pp 13-22.

Matheson, L.N., Ogden, L.D., Violette, K. and Schultz, K. (1985) 'Work hardening: occupational therapy in industrial rehabilitation', *American Journal of Occupational Therapy*, vol 39, no 5, pp 314-21.

McCluskey, A., Lovarini, M., Bennett, S., McKenna, K., Tooth, L. and Hoffman, T. (2005) 'What evidence exists for work-related injury prevention and management? Analysis of an occupational therapy evidence database (OTSeeker)', *British Journal of Occupational Therapy*, vol 68, no 10, pp 447-56.

Mechanic, D. (1995) 'Sociological dimensions of illness behaviour', *Social Science and Medicine*, vol 41, no 9, pp 1207-16.

Miles, M.B. and Huberman, A.M. (1994) *Qualitative data analysis: An expanded sourcebook* (2nd edn) Thousand Oaks, CA: Sage Publications.

Mountain, G., Carman, S. and Ilott, I. (2001) *Work rehabilitation and occupational therapy. A review of the literature*, London: College of Occupational Therapists.

Neff, W.S. (1976) 'Assessing vocational potential', in H. Rusalem and D. Malikin (eds) *Contemporary vocational rehabilitation*, New York, NY: New York University Press, pp 103-16.

Newman, S., Steed, L. and Mulligan, K. (2004) 'Self-management interventions for chronic illness', *Lancet*, vol 364, pp 1523-37.

O'Halloran, D. (2002) 'An historical overview of Australia's largest and oldest provider of vocational rehabilitation – CRS Australia', *Work*, vol 19, no 3, pp 211-18.

People Management (2004) 'UK is close to the top of the EU long-term sick list', *People Management,* vol 10, no 8, p 1. [Cited in: Chartered Institute of Personnel and Development (2004) Recovery, rehabilitation and retention: Maintaining a productive workforce. London: CIPD]

Perron, J. and McKay, M. (1997) 'Current models and trends in work practice service delivery', in J. Pratt and K. Jacobs (eds) *Work practice: International perspectives*, Oxford: Butterworth Heinemann.

Petrie, K.J., Weinman, J., Sharpe, N. and Buckley, J. (1996) 'Role of patients' view of their illness in predicting return to work and functioning after myocardial infarction: longitudinal study', *British Medical Journal,* vol 312, pp 1191-4.

Pratt, J. and Jacobs, K. (1997) (eds) *Work practice: International perspectives*, Oxford: Butterworth Heinemann.

Public Accounts Committee (2010) *First report: Support to incapacity benefits claimants through Pathways to Work*, London: The Stationery Office. www.publications.parliament.uk/pa/cm201011/cmselect/cmpubacc/404/40402.htm, accessed 15 January 2010.

Repper, J. and Perkins, R. (2003) *Social inclusion and recovery: A model for mental health practice*, Edinburgh: Ballière Tindall.

Ross, J. (2006) 'Meeting the challenge by mapping the curriculum: what do we learn about rehabilitation for work?', Paper presentation at the 14th Congress of the World Federation of Occupational Therapists, Sydney, Australia, 23-28 July.

Ross, J. (2007) *Occupational therapy and vocational rehabilitation*, East Sussex, Chichester: Wiley.

Ross, J. (2008) 'Understanding vocational rehabilitation: a cross-sector perspective using case study methodology', Unpublished PhD thesis, University of Kent at Canterbury.

Shaw, L. and Polatajko, H. (2002) 'An application of the occupational competence model to organizing factors associated with work', *Canadian Journal of Occupational Therapy*, vol 69, no 3, pp 158-67.

Shrey, D.E. and Hursh, N.C. (1999) 'Workplace disability management: international trends and perspectives', *Journal of Occupational Rehabilitation*, vol 9, no 1, pp 45-59.

Strong, S., Baptiste, S. and Salvatori, P. (2003) 'Learning from today's clinicians in vocational practice to educate tomorrow's therapists', *Canadian Journal of Occupational Therapy*, vol 70, no 1, pp 11-20.

Sullivan, M.J., Stanish, W., Waite, H., Sullivan, M. and Tripp, D.A. (1998) 'Catastrophizing, pain and disability in patients with soft-tissue injuries', *Pain*, vol 77, no 3, pp 253-60.

TUC (Trades Union Congress) (2002) *Rehabilitation and retention: What works is what matters*, London: TUC, www.tuc.org.uk

TUC (2007) 'Real, but oh so slow, progress on long hours', Press Release, 21 February, www.tuc.org.uk/work_life/tuc-12970-f0.cfm, accessed 24 February 2007.

United Kingdom Rehabilitation Council (2009) *Rehabilitation standards v1.0*, London: United Kingdom Rehabilitation Council.

Vocational Rehabilitation Association (2006) 'Recognising and accrediting education and training provision for the vocational rehabilitation professional', in *The way forward: A consultation paper*, Glasgow: Vocational Rehabilitation Association.

Vocational Rehabilitation Association (2007) *Standards of practice for vocational rehabilitation*, Glasgow: Vocational Rehabilitation Association.

Verbeek, J.H. (2006) 'How can doctors help their patients return to work?', *Public Library of Science: Medicine*, vol 3, no 3, p e88, published online March 28 available at: http://sciencestage.com/uploads/text/F4K4tiAAENyrWxNSnXzA.pdf

Waddell, G. and Aylward, M. (2005) *The scientific and conceptual basis of incapacity benefits*, London: The Stationery Office.

Waddell, G. and Burton, A.K. (2004) *Concepts of rehabilitation for the management of common mental health problems*, London: The Stationery Office.

Waddell, G. and Burton, A.K. (2006) *Is work good for your health and well-being?*, London: The Stationery Office.

Wehman, P. and Kreutzer, J.S. (1990) *Vocational rehabilitation for persons with traumatic brain injury*, Rockville, MD: Aspen Publishers.

Williams, R.M. and Westmorland, M. (2002) 'Perspectives on workplace disability management: a review of the literature', *Work,* vol 19, no 1, pp 87-93.

Wright, M., Beardwell, C. and Marsden, S. (2005) *Availability of rehabilitation services in the UK: A research study for the Association of British Insurers*, Reading: Greenstreet Berman Ltd, www.abi.org.uk/Publications/Availability_of_Rehabilitation_Services_in_the_UK1.aspx

Young (2010) *Common sense common safety*, London: The Cabinet Office.

SEVEN

The changing profile of incapacity claimants

Christina Beatty and Steve Fothergill

Introduction

Incapacity claimants are the single largest group of working-age benefit claimants in the UK. Even in the wake of the post-2008 recession, they outnumber the unemployed on Jobseeker's Allowance (JSA) by around one million and lone parents in receipt of Income Support by around two million. A total of 2.6 million adults of working age were out of the labour market on incapacity benefits in 2010 – 7% of the entire working-age population.

A sound understanding of just who makes up the stock of incapacity claimants, and why, is clearly important. Not least, this information is potentially helpful in trying to bring the numbers down. It is the government's stated intention to reduce the number claiming incapacity benefits by one million by 2016 (DWP, 2006, 2008) and there are a growing number of locally based initiatives that aim to help incapacity claimants back into work.

This chapter helps to fill the information gap by looking at how the profile of incapacity claimants has changed over the past decade. It does so primarily by drawing on survey evidence from one particular town, Barrow-in-Furness, where the incapacity claimant rate is especially high and where, uniquely, detailed survey data is available for two points in time. The chapter focuses in particular on the changing profile of the *men* claiming incapacity benefits but it also draws comparisons with the women claiming incapacity benefits.

As the chapter explains, the profile of incapacity claimants in Barrow-in-Furness is likely to be shared by many other older industrial areas. The radical changes in the composition of the stock of male incapacity claimants, identified in Barrow, therefore have important implications for welfare-to-work initiatives across Britain as a whole.

The next part of the chapter provides a brief introduction to incapacity benefits and the 'hidden unemployment' debate. This is followed by a short description of Barrow-in-Furness and the two surveys. The main body of the chapter then presents key findings. The final part sets out an explanation for the substantial changes that can be observed and the implications for public policy.

Incapacity benefits: a brief introduction

Incapacity benefits are paid to men and women of working age (that is 16-64 for men, 16-59 for women) who are out of work but deemed too ill or disabled to be required to look for work.[1] This differentiates them sharply from the claimant unemployed in receipt of JSA, who are required to look for work as a condition of benefit receipt. These two groups of benefit claimants are mutually exclusive: it is not possible to claim incapacity benefits and JSA at the same time.

The headline national total of 2.6 million incapacity claimants is actually made up of four groups:

- *Incapacity Benefit recipients.* In 2010, these men and women made up around half the total. Incapacity Benefit (IB) dates back to 1995, when it replaced Invalidity Benefit. IB is not means-tested except for a small number of post-2001 claimants with significant pension income.
- *Incapacity claimants who fail to qualify for Incapacity Benefit itself because they have insufficient National Insurance (NI) credits.* The government counts these men and women as IB claimants but most of these 'NI credits-only' claimants actually receive means-tested Income Support (IS), usually with a disability premium. They account for a further quarter of the national total, though a higher proportion of women than men.
- *Severe Disablement Allowance (SDA) recipients.* SDA is paid to pre-2001 claimants with a high level of disability and a poor NI contributions record. They account for around 10%. SDA is closed to new claimants.
- *Employment and Support Allowance (ESA) claimants.* ESA replaced IB (including the NI credits-only variety) for new claimants in October 2008. The intention is that between 2010 and 2013 all existing IB and SDA claimants will be gradually moved over to ESA, subject to the appropriate medical test. Eventually, therefore, ESA will account for all incapacity claimants.

The gatekeepers determining access to incapacity benefits are medical practitioners – in the first instance the claimant's own GP, but for claims beyond six months doctors working on behalf of the government agency Jobcentre Plus. In theory, to qualify for incapacity benefits a person must be unfit for work. In practice, the tests applied by Jobcentre Plus assess ability to undertake certain basic physical tasks rather than an inability to do all kinds of work in all circumstances. A new medical test – the Work Capability Assessment – was introduced in 2008 alongside ESA. Early experience with the new test is that it disqualifies a higher proportion of potential claimants, and as the existing stock of IB claimants is called in for re-testing this can be expected to have an important effect on benefit numbers. Nevertheless, many men and women have picked up injuries over the course of their working life, and there is the effect of simply getting older. On top of this, mental health problems such as stress and depression are quite widespread. In practice, therefore, many of the non-employed with health problems or disabilities are able to qualify for incapacity benefits rather than unemployment benefits.

In most circumstances, there is also a financial incentive to do so. IB (and its equivalent within ESA) is mostly not means-tested, unlike JSA, which is means-tested on the basis of household income and savings for everyone after six months and for most claimants from day one. This means that other sources of household income (a partner's earnings or a small pension, for example) are not deducted from an individual's IB entitlement as they would be for JSA. IS with a disability premium is also worth more than IS on its own. Additionally, there is also no requirement to 'sign on' every fortnight and to look for work as there is with JSA.

These differences in benefit rules, the large increase in the number of IB claimants since the late 1970s, and the concentration of IB claimants in many of the weakest labour markets across Britain have all fuelled the argument that incapacity benefits hide substantial unemployment. In studies of labour market adjustment in the UK coalfields (Beatty and Fothergill, 1996; Beatty et al, 2007a) we found that the main response to job loss was a withdrawal of men from the labour market into 'permanent sickness' rather than a rise in recorded unemployment. This led us to conclude that incapacity benefits hide the true scale of unemployment. Subsequently, we estimated that as many as one million incapacity claimants should be regarded as 'hidden unemployed' in that they might reasonably be expected to have been in work in a genuinely fully employed economy (see, for instance, Beatty and Fothergill, 2005).

Our view that job losses, rather than an underlying deterioration in health, underpin much of the four-fold increase in the number of incapacity claimants since the 1970s is supported by evidence from a number of other studies (for example, Armstrong, 1999; MacKay, 1999; Webster, 2002; Webster et al, 2010). An alternative but not necessarily incompatible view is that the rise in incapacity numbers reflects the deterioration of relative wages for low-skill (Nickell and Quintini, 2003, Bell and Smith, 2004). In the United States, a similar link is often established between falling labour demand, low wages and rising disability claims (see, for example, Black et al, 2002; Autor and Duggan, 2003).

Despite the fact that incapacity numbers are vastly higher than a generation ago, benefits data from the Department for Work and Pensions (DWP) provides surprisingly few insights into the changing profile of claimants. It tells us that the over-50s account for around 45% of the total, but that this proportion has declined slightly in recent years. It tells us that claimants are remaining on incapacity benefits for longer – around half have been claiming for five years or more. The benefits data also tells us that a higher proportion of claimants are now women – among the under-60s, the ratio between men and women is now 52:48, compared with 60:40 in the mid 1980s.[2] In addition, it tells us that 'mental and behavioural problems' now account for a higher proportion of incapacity claims, mainly at the expense of claims based on musculoskeletal problems.

But beyond this basic information, little has hitherto been known about the changing profile of incapacity claimants. Even the government's otherwise admirable Labour Force Survey is of limited help because it under-counts the overall number of incapacity claimants by as much as three quarters of a million, compared with benefit records, and the under-counting is particularly marked for the large group of NI credits-only IB claimants. This is why the local survey evidence, presented here, is so helpful.

A case study: Barrow-in-Furness

Barrow-in-Furness, in Cumbria in north-west England, is a relatively isolated town, more than 40 miles from the nearest significant urban area (around Lancaster). It sits at the end of a peninsula with the sea to the west and south and the sparsely populated fells of the Lake District to the north. This means that Barrow is an essentially self-contained labour market, with only modest commuting flows in and out of the area.

Perhaps more than any other UK town of comparable size – the district has a population of 70,000 – Barrow has traditionally been dominated by a single industrial employer. This is its shipyard, dating back to the 19th century, which has long specialised in major defence contracts and in submarines in particular. It was here that Britain's four Trident missile submarines were built in the 1980s and 1990s. At its peak, the shipyard accounted for nearly 70% of all male employment in the town, but as the Trident construction programme came to an end some 9,000 jobs were shed from the shipyard.

In Barrow, the combination of job loss and physical isolation might have been expected to lead to rising unemployment. But this did not happen. Claimant unemployment in the town (that is, the number claiming what is now JSA) fell almost continuously between 1993 and 2008. There was some growth in alternative employment, but nothing like on the scale needed to plug the gap left by the disappearance of so many shipbuilding jobs.

Barrow does, however, have one of the highest incapacity claimant rates in the country. This is illustrated in Table 7.1, which shows the 20 local authority districts in Britain with the highest share of the working-age population claiming incapacity benefits. Barrow comes 17th on this list (out of nearly 400 districts) with a rate of 11.5%. Like Barrow, virtually all the top 20 are industrial districts in the North, Scotland and Wales. In contrast, in extensive parts of southern England

Table 7.1: Incapacity claimant rate, top 20 districts, Britain, February 2009

		% of working age
1.	Merthyr Tydfil	16.1
2.	Blaenau Gwent	15.7
3.	Neath Port Talbot	15.2
4.	Rhondda Cynon Taf	14.5
5.	Caerphilly	13.7
6.	Glasgow	13.5
7.	Knowsley	13.1
8.	Blackpool	12.9
9.	Liverpool	12.9
10.	Inverclyde	12.8
11.	Bridgend	12.6
12.	Stoke on Trent	12.1
13.	Burnley	12.1
14.	Hartlepool	12.0
15.	Carmarthenshire	12.0
16.	Blackburn	11.7
17.	BARROW-IN-FURNESS	11.5
18.	Barnsley	11.5
19.	Dundee	11.5
20.	Torfaen	11.5

Sources: DWP (2009); ONS (2009)

the incapacity claimant rate is typically 3-4%, with rates as low as 2% recorded in some districts.

The first survey of incapacity claimants in Barrow was carried out in the autumn of 1999. This covered 329 non-employed men of working age, of whom 183 were IB claimants. The survey was undertaken in four representative wards within the district, selected on the basis of levels of non-employment. Individuals were contacted via door-to-door visits, and interviewed in their own home by professional survey staff. The results of this survey are reported in Beatty and Fothergill (2002).

The second survey was carried out in two phases in the final part of 2006 and spring of 2007. This covered 999 incapacity claimants in all, of whom 488 were men. The survey took place in 25 postcode areas spread randomly across the whole district. Names and addresses of claimants were obtained directly from the DWP, which had agreed to support a wider national research project to which the Barrow survey contributed. The individuals were again interviewed in their own home by professional survey staff. The results of this second survey are reported in Beatty et al (2007b).

Both surveys used a tightly structured questionnaire covering aspects of work history, skills, health, job aspirations, training needs, benefits and household circumstances. Several key questions were identical in the two surveys. Each interview typically lasted 15-30 minutes. Because of differences in methods the two surveys were not absolutely precisely comparable. On the other hand, neither survey encountered a significant opt-out rate on the doorstep. With the proviso that very small differences between the findings of the two surveys should not be given any weight, the two datasets are nevertheless likely to be broadly representative of incapacity claimants in Barrow and comparable through time.

The changing profile of men on incapacity benefits

The Barrow data allows the 183 male IB claimants in the 1999 survey to be compared with the 488 male IB claimants in the 2007 survey.

In terms of age, 52% of the male incapacity claimants in the 2007 survey were aged between 55 and 64, compared with 55% in this age group in 1999. What is significant here is not the slight reduction in the proportion of over-55s, which is in line with national trends but too small to be given any weight, but the fact that by 2007 around three quarters of the over-55s who were IB claimants back in 1999 would have reached 65 and thereby dropped off incapacity benefits on to state pension. Through the ageing process alone there must therefore have been substantial turnover in the stock of IB claimants. What happened in Barrow was that the 1999 cohort of older male IB claimants was by 2007 largely replaced by a different cohort, as existing claimants grew older and new over-55s joined the stock.

The overall stock of male IB claimants may not therefore have been getting any older, but in Barrow at least they have been out of work for much longer. This is illustrated in Table 7.2, which shows the length of time since the claimant's last regular paid job. In 1999 only around one in eight men had been out of work for 10 years or more. By 2007, this had risen to nearly half. Not all of this long duration out of work need necessarily have been on incapacity benefits – initially some claimed unemployment benefits, for example – but 40% said they had been claiming IB for at least 10 years. The conventional view,

Table 7.2: Male IB claimants in Barrow: length of time since last regular paid job

	1999 (%)	2007 (%)
Less than 2 years	10	8
2-5 years	27	22
5-10 years	49	22
10 years or more	13	46
Never had job	1	3
	100	100

Source: Barrow surveys

at least among labour market economists, is that the employability of an individual declines with rising duration out of work, in which case Barrow's stock of male IB claimants has become markedly less employable now than in the late 1990s.

A further key indicator of employability is qualifications. Table 7.3 shows selected qualifications held by Barrow's male IB claimants. What needs to be kept in mind here is that many people have more than one qualification (so the columns do not add to 100) and there are many different types of qualification. The striking figure here is the large share of male IB claimants who had no formal qualifications at all. Even more shocking, this proportion rose from 38% in 1999 to 53% in 2007. This is the opposite of what might have been expected because over

Table 7.3: Male IB claimants in Barrow: selected qualifications

	1999 (%)	2007 (%)
Degree	2	3
'O' level/CSE/GCSE	24	22
NVQ/ONC/OND/HNC/HND*	10	10
Craft apprenticeship	37	21
No formal qualifications	38	53

Notes: * National Vocational Qualifications/Ordinary National Certificate/Ordinary National Diploma/Higher National Certificate/Higher National Diploma
Source: Barrow surveys

this period a group of older men with no formal qualifications, who mostly entered the labour market in the 1950s when qualifications were deemed less essential, finally reached retirement age. As they did so, they were replaced in the workforce by a younger generation of new workers with more education and training. As a result, across the UK as a whole, the share of working-age adults with no formal qualifications has been falling. Barrow's male IB claimants appear to buck this well-established trend. The rise of claimants with no formal qualifications is also matched by a fall in the share that had served a craft apprenticeship – down by nearly half since 1999.

Table 7.4 deals with the occupational background of male IB claimants. These statistics are based on what men called their 'usual occupation' and the various jobs have been grouped into four broad categories. Professionals account for very few IB claimants – in Barrow or elsewhere in Britain. Manual workers dominate the figures for both years – they accounted for 76% in 1999 and 81% in 2007. The 'other manual' category includes plant and machine operatives, drivers, shop workers, labourers and those providing routine personal

Table 7.4: Male IB claimants in Barrow: occupational background

	1999 (%)	2007 (%)
Professional	2	3
Other white-collar	22	16
Skilled manual	49	31
Other manual	27	50
	100	100

Source: Barrow surveys

services. This category alone accounted for half the men claiming IB in 2007, and the 'other manual' category grew substantially after 1999, largely at the expense of skilled manual workers.

On balance, therefore, the stock of male IB claimants remained primarily manual but shifted towards the lower-skill categories. Even so, these men were rarely lacking in substantial work experience, even if it was receding into the past. Among the 2007 claimants, 40% had worked in their last job for 20 years or more, and a further 20% for between 10 and 20 years.

The reasons why individuals leave a job may be complex. Sometimes there is a single, clear-cut reason. On other occasions, job loss is the result of the interaction of a number of factors – for example, cuts in a firm's workforce combined with personal ill health, domestic responsibilities and maybe even a bullying or unsympathetic boss. The two surveys asked men to identify the *principal* reason for leaving their last regular paid job. Table 7.5 shows the responses.

A striking feature here is the importance of illness or disability as the trigger of job loss among the 2007 claimants, cited by around

Table 7.5: Male IB claimants in Barrow: principal reasons for job loss

	1999 (%)	2007 (%)
Compulsory severance*	27	14
Voluntary – redundancy/retirement	23	4
Voluntary – other reasons	9	3
Illness or injury	40	78
Other	1	2
	100	100

Note: *Compulsory redundancy, dismissal, end of contract

Source: Barrow surveys

three quarters of the total. By comparison, other factors were far less significant. Compulsory severance, for example, accounted for only 14% and voluntary redundancy or retirement for only 4%. At least as striking, however, is the change through time. The 1999 survey asked exactly the same question and at that time illness or injury was the primary reason for job loss in only 40% of cases, while compulsory and voluntary redundancy together accounted for half. Bearing in mind that at least some of the men who were claiming incapacity benefits in 1999 were still claimants in 2007, the data on the causes of job loss indicates that since the late 1990s there have been radical changes in the reasons why male IB claimants' last jobs came to an end. Formerly redundancy was dominant; now it is overwhelmingly ill health.

On the other hand, the evidence does not support the view that on average the health of male IB claimants is any worse now than in the late 1990s. Table 7.6 combines the responses to several health questions that were again identical in the two surveys. The data deals with claimant's own assessment of the influence of health on their ability to work. A degree of self-reported health limitation is nearly universal, but in both years only a third said they 'can't do any work'. Overall, there is little evidence of a change through time.

Table 7.6: Male IB claimants in Barrow: self-assessment of influence of health on ability to work

	1999 (%)	2007 (%)
'Can't do any work'	34	37
'A lot' of limitation	39	32
Some limitation	24	26
No limitation	3	5
	100	100

Source: Barrow surveys

Table 7.7 deals with job aspirations. This, too, combines the answers to several questions that were the same in the two surveys. The first line presents the responses to the question 'would you like a job?' There are two extremely important observations here. First, in 2007 the

Table 7.7: Male IB claimants in Barrow: job aspirations

	1999 (%)	2007 (%)
Would like a job	64	18
Looked after last job ended	30	13
Looking now	4	8
Thinks there is a realistic chance of ever getting one	8	5

Source: Barrow surveys

proportion of male IB claimants saying they would like a job was just 18%. Second, the proportion wanting work slipped from no less than 64% in 1999. Barrow's male IB claimants are now, it would appear, a demotivated group with few aspirations to work and their detachment from the labour market has increased sharply in recent years.

The second line in the table shows the proportion who looked for work after their last job ended. This was not large, and the share was again well down on 1999. The declining proportion looking for work at the time of job loss is consistent with the rising proportion who said they lost their last job principally for reasons of ill health.

The third line shows the proportion who said they were presently looking for work. This is below 10%, though the number of active jobseekers appears to have increased slightly since 1999. It is worth noting here that there are often fears among IB claimants that to be seen to look for work would bring their status as an IB claimant into question. ESA, which is now progressively replacing IB, for the first time introduces an element of conditionality similar to that already in place for JSA. For all but the most severely ill, this is to undertake activities to 'progress towards work', which may be rehabilitation, retraining or voluntary work as well as job search.

The final line of the table refers to those who would like a job and think there is a realistic chance of getting one. The figures show little optimism.

What about women?

The Barrow-in-Furness surveys do not provide data on women for the earlier year but for the later year (2007) information on 511 women on incapacity benefits is available on the same basis as for men. The women are on average a marginally younger group, reflecting the fact that women move on to a state pension five years earlier, but in most other respects they look remarkably similar to Barrow's male IB claimants:

- 38% of women had been claiming incapacity benefits for at least 10 years (compared with 40% of men);
- 52% of women on IB had no formal qualifications (compared with 53% of men)
- 47% of women on IB had not had regular paid employment for at least 10 years (46% for men);
- 79% of the women worked in manual jobs (81% for men);
- Only 32% of the women said they 'can't do any work' (37% for men);
- Only 19% of the women said they would like a job (18% for men);
- 93% of the women who said they did not want a job gave ill health, injury or disability as the main reason (93% for men).

What this information tells us is that the men and women who claim incapacity benefits occupy much the same segment of the labour market, and a relatively lowly segment too. They are a predominantly poorly qualified group, with mainly low-grade manual experience, and have often not worked for many years.

The marginalisation of the least healthy

The survey evidence on incapacity claimants provides important insights into the way the contemporary labour market works.

Let us begin with the changing profile of the male IB client group. What the evidence from Barrow shows is that, over time, this group has become substantially more disengaged from the labour market and, as a result, looks far harder to move back towards employment. The key points in this respect are the increase in the share of claimants who have been on incapacity benefits for a very long time, the increase in the share with no formal qualifications, the increase in the share with low-skill manual experience, and the sharp decline in the share saying they would like a job.

In Barrow's case, the starting point in explaining these trends is almost certainly the redundancies from the town's shipyard. These job losses mostly occurred during the early and mid-1990s. Many of the unemployed shipyard workers moved onto IB rather than unemployment benefits because they were financially better off doing so and because they had sufficient health problems or disabilities to allow them to access incapacity benefits. In 1999, when the first survey was conducted, it therefore found a large group of often skilled men who had been made redundant (either compulsorily or voluntarily, though the distinction can be blurred when firms are shedding labour) and had not lost residual aspirations to work.

By 2007 many of this group of ex-shipyard workers had dropped off incapacity benefits – some back into work no doubt, but very many simply on to state pension at age 65. However, with a continuing imbalance in the Barrow labour market, with the local demand for labour still running well behind the potential local labour supply, it was inevitable that some individuals would continue to be squeezed out. What appears to have happened is that the men who have been squeezed out more recently are those least able or least willing to keep a foothold in the local labour market. These are typically the least skilled, the least healthy and (to some extent, no doubt) the least motivated.

Many of the newer IB claimants lost their last job because of ill health rather than redundancy. In a difficult labour market like Barrow they then find it nigh on impossible to return to work even if they want to do so – and many are pragmatic enough to not even bother trying. More of the newer IB claimants are also women and, in so far as men and women often compete for the same jobs, a difficult local labour market for men will through normal competitive processes produce a difficult local labour market for women as well. There is clear evidence in another study (Beatty et al, 2009) of this transmission of job loss and benefit claims from men to women. In Barrow's case the male ex-shipyard workers may have shunned jobs that they saw as 'women's work', but their sons will often have had little choice but to compete for work in sectors such as retailing, catering, hospitals and call centres.

The effect of lengthening durations on incapacity benefits is by itself likely to sap the enthusiasm of many to re-engage with the labour market. Long-term IB claimants will in many cases have adjusted their lifestyle and aspirations to fit with the diminished job opportunities they perceive as available to them, lowering their standards of consumption to fit with ongoing benefit dependency. Their 'fitness to work' may also decline as despondency sets in and disabilities worsen with age. An initial willingness to consider new employment is thus gradually replaced by a complete detachment from the world of work, rationalised in terms of largely insurmountable health obstacles.

So although the number of incapacity claimants in a town such as Barrow has fallen modestly since its peak in the early 2000s, the composition and outlook of this group have undergone a transformation. The skilled male craftsman, forced out by redundancy and still hankering after employment, is disappearing. His place has been taken by the poorly qualified, low-skill manual worker in poor health, whose alternative would at best be unrewarding work at or close to the national minimum wage. His place has also been taken by rising numbers of equally poorly qualified, low-skill women in poor health.

A key question, of course, is the extent to which the survey findings from Barrow can be generalised to other areas. In the absence of survey data at two points in time for other areas, it is not possible to give a definitive answer. On the other hand, the circumstances in Barrow are not unique. Just as Barrow experienced massive redundancies from its shipyard during the 1990s, many coalmining areas, steel towns and other centres of heavy industry were hit by large job losses in the 1980s and 1990s. In just about all these places, a big increase in the incapacity claimant rate was one of the main results, and these places continue to dominate the list of districts with the highest incapacity claimant rates in Britain.

Moreover, just as with the passage of time many of Barrow's shipyard workers will have passed out of the incapacity numbers and on to state pensions, the same will be true of ex-miners, ex-steelworkers and other victims of the industrial restructuring of the last part of the 20th century. There is reason to believe, therefore, that in the same way that male incapacity claimants in Barrow are becoming dominated by the least qualified, least healthy and (probably) the least motivated, the same process will be at work in other older industrial areas. In this way, an initially qualified and motivated group of IB claimants stands every chance of being gradually eroded, to be replaced by men (and women) whose ability or willingness to maintain a foothold in the labour market is more questionable.

If this is indeed the case, it makes the task of bringing down the numbers claiming incapacity benefits a lot harder. A decade ago, the relatively high level of skills among IB claimants and the residual motivation to work of many suggested that if sufficient jobs could be created in the right places this should in itself begin to bring some of them back into work. Now, by virtue of their poor health, low skills and long duration on benefit, the vast majority of the men and women claiming IB are unlikely to be employers' first choice to fill vacancies. Accordingly, expanding the demand for labour is on its own unlikely to be enough to bring many of these men and women back into work.

The last phase of the long economic boom up to 2008 illustrates this point. Once claimant unemployment had, by the early 2000s, been brought down to historically low levels, it might have been expected that further job creation would erode the numbers on incapacity benefits. In practice, although the IB numbers did fall by 150,000-200,000, a surge in the number of migrant workers, especially from central and eastern Europe, accounted for much of the rise in employment. Most incapacity claimants were neither sufficiently engaged with the labour market nor sufficiently attractive to potential employers.

Additional demand for labour remains an essential part of the jigsaw, without which it is hard to see opportunities becoming available for many men and women currently outside the labour market, but the evidence suggests that this will need to be complemented by labour market activation measures targeted at IB claimants. These need to include retraining, remotivation and, where appropriate, physical and mental rehabilitation programmes. It probably also needs the financial rewards for returning to work to be worthwhile, which is not easily achievable in areas where low-skill workers command only low wages.

The package of reforms to incapacity benefits that the UK government began to introduce from 2008 onwards does include these elements. The national roll-out of the Pathways to Work initiative combined access to training, rehabilitation and wage top-ups for those entering low-paid employment. The new ESA will eventually require most incapacity claimants to engage in activity to prepare for work.

The trouble is that these policies now look to be 'too little, too late'. The favourable labour market conditions of the pre-2008 era have receded for the foreseeable future. The newly unemployed, on JSA, are more likely to be employers' first choice because of their recent work experience and better health. Recession will have moved incapacity claimants further back in the queue for jobs.

The welfare reforms designed for a buoyant labour market therefore appear increasingly anachronistic. Above all, as the existing stock of IB claimants is called in for new, tougher medical tests and (if they qualify for ESA) for compulsory work-focused interviews and to draw up plans to progress towards work, they will have legitimate cause for complaint. As the evidence presented here shows, this is a group that mostly faces formidable obstacles to employment – poor qualifications, low-grade work experience and a long time out of work, as well as poor health or disability. They might reasonably argue that in the post-recession world their chances of finding work are just about nil. That so many of Britain's incapacity claimants live in the weaker local labour markets up and down the country only adds to the validity of their concerns.

In the context of wider concerns about the effective management of health at work, as considered in this volume, the group who make up incapacity claimants put into sharp relief the complicated dynamics of health issues, job quality and local labour market opportunities. This lends urgency to measures aimed at increasing demand for labour and improving job quality to help keep people with health conditions in the workplace wherever possible so as not to swell the already large ranks of the marginalised least healthy dependent on state benefits.

Notes

[1] Men and women over state pension age who continue in employment can claim incapacity benefits for a short period if they are temporarily ill or incapacitated, but the numbers doing so are very small.

[2] Women move across on to state pension earlier than men (60 rather than 65 in 2010), so including 60- to 64-year-olds the total number of men claiming incapacity benefits (1.5 million) continues to outstrip the number of women (1.1 million).

Further reading

Beatty, C. and Fothergill, S. (2005) 'The diversion from "unemployment" to "sickness" across British regions and districts', *Regional Studies*, vol 39, no 7, pp 837-54, www.informaworld.com/smpp/content~db=all~content=a747359804.

Beatty, C., Fothergill, S., Houston, D., Powell, R. and Sissons, P. (2009) *Women on incapacity benefits*, Sheffield: *Centre for Regional, Economic and Social Research*, Sheffield Hallam University with Department of Geography, University of Dundee, www.shu.ac.uk/_assets/pdf/cresr-women-on-IB.pdf

DWP (Department for Work and Pensions) (2010) *Universal credit: Welfare that works*, London: The Stationery Office, www.dwp.gov.uk/docs/universal-credit-full-document.pdf.

Lindsey, C. and Houston D. (2011) 'Fit for purpose? Welfare reform and challenges for health and labour market policy in the UK', *Environment and Planning A*, vol 43, no 3, pp 703-21, www.envplan.com/epa/fulltext/a43/a43442.pdf

Policy Studies, 'Fit for work? Health, employability and challenges for the UK welfare reform agenda', vol 31, no 2, March 2010, Special issue, www.informaworld.com/smpp/title~db=all~content=g919727333

References

Armstrong, D. (1999) 'Hidden male unemployment in Northern Ireland', *Regional Studies*, vol 33, no 6, pp 499-512.

Autor, D.H. and Duggan, M.G. (2003) 'The rise in the disability rolls and the decline in unemployment', *Quarterly Journal of Economics*, vol 118, no 1, pp 157-206.

Beatty, C. and Fothergill, S. (1996) 'Labour market adjustment in areas of chronic industrial decline: the case of the UK coalfields', *Regional Studies*, vol 30, no 7, pp 627-40.

Beatty, C. and Fothergill, S. (2002) 'Hidden unemployment among men: a case study', *Regional Studies*, vol 36, no 8, pp 811-23.

Beatty, C. and Fothergill, S. (2005) 'The diversion from "unemployment" to "sickness" across British regions and districts', *Regional Studies*, vol 39, no 7, pp 837-54.

Beatty, C., Fothergill, S. and Powell, R. (2007a) 'Twenty years on: has the economy of the UK coalfields recovered?', *Environment and Planning A*, vol 39, no 7, pp 1654-75.

Beatty, C., Fothergill, S., Gore, T. and Powell, R. (2007b) *Barrow's incapacity claimants*, Sheffield: CRESR, Sheffield Hallam University.

Beatty, C., Fothergill, S., Houston, D., Powell, R. and Sissons, P. (2009) *Women on incapacity benefits*, Sheffield: *Centre for Regional, Economic and Social Research*, Sheffield Hallam University with Department of Geography, University of Dundee.

Bell, B. and Smith, J. (2004) *Health, disability insurance and labour force participation*, Working Paper No 218, London: Bank of England.

Black, D., Kermit, D. and Sanders, S. (2002) 'The impact of economic conditions on participation in disability programs: evidence from the coal boom and bust', *American Economic Review*, vol 92, no 1, pp 27-50.

DWP (Department for Work and Pensions) (2006) *A new deal for welfare: Empowering people to work*, Cm 6730 , London: The Stationery Office, www.dwp.gov.uk/docs/a-new-deal-for-welfare-empowering-people-to-work-full-document.pdf

DWP (2008) *No one written off: Reforming welfare to reward responsibility*, Cm 7363, London: The Stationery Office, www.dwp.gov.uk/docs/noonewrittenoff-complete.pdf

MacKay, R. (1999) 'Work and nonwork: a more difficult labour market', *Environment and Planning A*, vol 31, no 11, pp 487-502.

Nickell, S. and Quintini, G. (2003) 'The recent performance of the UK labour market', *Oxford Review of Economic Policy*, vol 18, no 2, pp 202-20.

Webster, D. (2002) 'Unemployment: how official statistics distort analysis and policy, and why', *Radical Statistics*, vol 79/80, Summer/ Winter, pp 96-127.

Webster, D., Arnott, J., Brown, J., Turok, I., Mitchell, R. and Macdonald, E.B. (2010) 'Falling Incapacity Benefit claims in a former industrial city: policy impacts or labour market improvement?', *Policy Studies*, vol 31, no 2 pp 163-85.

EIGHT

Reconstructing the self and social identity: new interventions for returning long-term Incapacity Benefit recipients to work

David Wainwright, Elaine Wainwright, Rachel Black and Susan Kenyon

Introduction

Returning one million Incapacity Benefit (IB) recipients to work by 2015 is high on the UK government's disability reform agenda. Several interventions have been piloted in the Pathways to Work initiative and have proven moderately successful at returning *new* IB claimants to work. However, we know little about how they are experienced by *long-term* IB recipients.

This chapter presents evidence of the problems faced by long-term IB recipients and the limited effectiveness of current interventions to support their return to work. We undertook qualitative interviews with 12 long-term IB recipients who had used return-to-work interventions provided by a council in southern England. This council was among the first to provide a service targeted specifically at long-term IB recipients, but it had limited success. Our interviews reveal the damage to self and social identity that often accompanies life on IB; the non-linear process of repairing this damage; the obstacles that impede return to work; and the limitations of 'off-the-shelf' interventions.

The chapter supports the conclusion that long-term IB recipients require bespoke and holistic rehabilitation to repair the damage to their self and social identity. Government policy emphasises the need for personalised care, but the mechanism for delivering rehabilitation may militate against this approach.

In 2008, the UK government replaced IB, paid to working-age people who are considered to be incapable of paid employment for medical reasons, with a new Employment Support Allowance (ESA)

(DWP, 2008). The reform reflects a policy debate about inappropriate uptake of IB, which led the government to set a target of one million IB recipients returned to work by 2015 (DWP, 2008, p 6). This might be addressed by reducing the inflow of recipients, or by increasing the outflow of long-term recipients off benefit and back into work. This chapter concerns the latter and more challenging approach.

We present evidence from a qualitative study of a programme designed to return long-term IB recipients to work. Our aim is not to present an evaluation, but to provide a rich account of the experiences of long-term IB recipients who chose to participate in the programme, in order to deepen our understanding of the nature of the problems they face and derive recommendations for policy initiatives that more adequately address their needs.

The genesis of IB reform

Between 1979 and 1995, the number of recipients of Invalidity Benefit (the precursor to IB) rose from 700,000 to 2.6 million, although the number has plateaued since (Waddell and Aylward, 2005). This increase is widely seen as a response to non-medical factors, including recession, restructuring and the tightening of unemployment benefits, leading to the conclusion that the benefit is being used by many who could work, as well as by those who are incapacitated by medical problems (Bambra, 2008). Thus, the concern for policymakers is partly a moral one that resonates with a long-standing political narrative about the 'deserving' and 'undeserving' poor (Katz, 1989; Fideler, 2005).

This concern is strengthened when the health problems of long-term IB recipients are examined. Only a quarter have severe medical conditions for which there is objective evidence of pathology. The remaining three quarters have less severe common health problems (Waddell and Burton, 2004; Waddell and Aylward, 2005), or medically unexplained symptoms (Page and Wessely, 2003) with diagnosis dependent on the patient's subjective description of symptoms. The absence of medical reasons for much long-term uptake of IB has fuelled calls for a 'stick-and-carrot' approach that will make long-term benefit uptake more difficult to sustain and provide stronger incentives to return to work, (Field, 2007). It is assumed that if employment is more attractive than life on benefits, recipients will choose to return to work. However, for many IB recipients paid employment has always been more lucrative than life on benefits (Wainwright, 2004), but there are psychosocial factors that make return to work difficult to achieve.

This has generated a second strand to the policy debate and it is to this psychosocial discourse that we now turn.

Psychosocial concepts

Uptake of IB is not simply the result of unmediated pathology; it is also influenced by a range of psychosocial factors, including the free will and agency of the individual (Leonard et al, 1999). Thus, understanding long-term uptake of IB, and the interventions required to ameliorate it, entails going beyond the biomedical model to consider the psychosocial processes that influence this form of illness behaviour (Mechanic, 1999; Young, 2004; Wainwright, 2008).

Many concepts can be brought to bear on this issue, for example, self-efficacy (Bandura, 1977, 1991), coping (Lazarus and Folkman, 1984), external locus of control (Rotter, 1975), learned helplessness (Abramson, 1978), rational choice theory (Heath, 1976), adaptation theory (Twaddle, 1973) and labelling theory (Becker, 1973). The categories we have applied are *self* and *social identity*. These were chosen because they offered the best fit with the themes that emerged from our data.

Self and social identity have a long history in psychological and sociological thought, particularly in the writings of William James (1892), Charles Horton Cooley (1981) and George Herbert Mead (1934). For these writers, the self refers to an inner awareness of subjectivity that is unique to an individual and cannot be directly known by others. Self comprises the sum of personal knowledge and experience by which we recognise ourselves as a particular human being with distinctive qualities and attributes (Field, 1974; Douglas, 1984) and by which the external world is interpreted (Wagner, 1970). Reflexivity, the capacity to reflect on the self as an object, in the same way that one reflects on others, is an essential aspect of selfhood. Key to this process is taking the role of the other and imagining how others might perceive and understand us (Mead, 1934, 1981).

Self has a potent effect on behaviour; it is the repository of internalised role expectations and ways of being in the world (McCall and Simmons, 1966). While self is relatively stable over time, it is also capable of change (Ball, 1972). Giddens (1991) has described the process of reflexive reconstruction of the self in which the individual reflects on the self and seeks to transform it. Although the self is constituted by reflection or reflexivity, internal views of self must be legitimated by others through social interaction, with real or imagined external legitimation incorporated into definitions of self (Burke, 1980). Self, although a highly individual and personal phenomenon, therefore, has a social character – how we think of ourselves is strongly influenced by how others respond to us in social interaction, and we reflexively seek out knowledge and experiences that will change our sense of self.

Social identity refers to what other people know about us, including not only our position in social hierarchies, and broad characteristics including age, gender and occupation, but also more intimate knowledge of personal characteristics and attributes. As with the self, social identity is a set of meanings attributed to someone by themselves and others; we attempt to manage our social identity by presenting the self to the world in a particular way, but identity is modified by the reactions of others who may make alternative attributions (Weinstein and Deutschberger, 1963; Gergen, 1971). We are able to take the role of the other and imagine how our self-identity will be interpreted and defined by others. Moreover, when others attribute characteristics to our identity, for example, intelligence or laziness, this may have consequences for the self, if we internalise their attribution and modify our definitions of the self. There is, therefore, a tension between the self and social identity as we struggle to maintain a positive sense of self and present it to the world, which in turn may contest or modify our social identity in ways that may have consequences for the self.

A key concept in mediating the relationship between self and social identity is stigma. For Erving Goffman, stigma is a social response to deviance, that is, it is a mechanism by which 'normal' members of society label individuals who have transgressed social norms (Goffman, 1968). In this sense, stigma marks out the individual as having a *spoiled identity*, for example, criminal, mental patient or, in this instance, the 'undeserving' benefit recipient. Stigma not only influences how others respond to the deviant, but may also be internalised by the individual giving rise to a new sense of selfhood:

> Those who have dealings with him fail to accord him the respect and regard which the un-contaminated aspects of his social identity have led him to anticipate extending and have led him to anticipate receiving; he echoes this denial by finding that some of his own attributes warrant it. (Goffman, 1968, p 19)

Crucially for Goffman, the process of stigmatisation does not simply entail society imposing a label on a passive subject; rather, it is a dynamic process in which the individual struggles to manage, for instance by attempting to conceal the stigma (*passing*) or minimising its significance (*covering*). Alternatively, the individual may band together with other members of his stigmatised group (the *in-group*) and lobby for better treatment by the normals. A less confrontational response is to take on normative beliefs about what constitutes '*good personal adjustment*', by adopting an identity that conforms to the perceptions of the *out-group* (the normals), and which minimises the disruptive effects of their deviance. Goffman sees this process as *phantom acceptance*, which may not be in the interests of the stigmatised individual:

> The nature of a 'good adjustment' is now apparent. It requires that the stigmatised individual cheerfully and unselfconsciously accepts himself as essentially the same as normals....The stigmatised individual is asked to act so as to imply neither that his burden is heavy nor that bearing it has made him different from us; at the same time he must keep himself at that remove from us which ensures our painlessly being able to confirm this belief about him. Put differently, he is advised to reciprocate naturally with an acceptance of him and us, an acceptance of him that we have not quite extended in the first place. A *phantom acceptance* is thus allowed to provide the base for a *phantom normalcy*. (Goffman, 1968, pp 147-8, emphasis in original)

Goffman's concerns about the normalising character of 'good adjustment' are particularly pertinent to initiatives that aim to return long-term IB recipients to work. Certainly, members of this group are frequently stigmatised as 'malingerers', and their participation in return to work initiatives arguably entails embracing a normative viewpoint on the nature of their problems and accepting employment opportunities that are often so marginal that they might well be construed as a form of phantom acceptance. Alternatively, it could be argued that exclusion from work is an even more damning fate and that initiatives that seek to reintegrate the individual into working life (even if the work is low status and poorly paid) are more progressive than simply leaving the individual on long-term incapacity benefits. Clearly, the project of repairing spoiled identity in order to facilitate return to work has profoundly political ramifications that must be considered when appraising the value of such schemes. We will return to this theme in our conclusion.

More fundamentally, this line of reasoning leads to a questioning of the assumption that paid employment has a positive impact on the self. The role of work in shaping selfhood and contributing to self-realisation is a prominent theme in the sociology of work (see Grint, 2005 for an overview of the main contributions to this debate). Since the advent of industrial capitalism, commentators have argued that while productive activity is central to human fulfilment and happiness, the specific form of paid employment can have negative consequences for self-realisation: 'For Ruskin, Carlyle, Morris, Hobhouse and even J.S. Mill and Marx, work *should*, but self-evidently did not, provide the material base for the self-development of all' (Grint, 2005, p 17, emphasis in original).

Thus, for Marx, productive activity was central to the human species being, providing intrinsic rewards by enabling workers to realise themselves through transformation of the world and yielding a sufficient surplus to support other creative and intellectual pursuits. However, the alienated and oppressive character of work under capitalism broke the link between production and self-realisation (Avineri, 1968); rather than a means of self-realisation, work was transformed into a profoundly dehumanising experience. From this perspective, return to work cannot be uncritically accepted as a panacea for the spoiled identity. Even so, whatever the consequences of paid employment are for the self and social identity, they are surely more positive than the consequences of long-term unemployment and incapacity.

This chapter explores damage to the self and social identity caused by the stigma of long-term uptake of IB, and the extent to which return-to-work interventions can repair the damage. First, we introduce the interventions that have been applied nationally and those that were the focus of our study.

Pathways to Work and the South East Opportunities for Work initiative

The Pathways to Work programme was central to the government's IB reforms, which aim to draw a distinction between those with severe physical impairment who are incapable of work and those with less severe illnesses who could return to work (DWP, 2006, 2008). Pathways will remain a central plank of government reforms until the new Work Programme is introduced, in summer 2011 (DWP, 2010). The Work Programme will replace existing employment schemes such as Pathways and is designed to support longer-term benefit customers into work. Later, we consider whether or not the Work Programme appears likely to include elements similar to our recommendations for policy initiatives designed to help long-term IB recipients. Pathways was piloted in three Jobcentre Plus districts in October 2003 and was rolled out nationally from April 2008. All new IB claimants are obliged to attend a work-focused interview (WFI) with an IB personal adviser.

Those with severe medical conditions are exempt from further WFIs, while others must attend up to five more. The remaining components of the Pathways programme are voluntary and include interventions to improve labour market readiness and opportunities, including a 'condition management programme', a 'Return-to-Work Credit' of £40 per week for a year and 'in-work support', which can include mentoring, occupational health support and an aftercare service.

Where the Pathways pilots were not operating 29.7% of *new* claimants returned to work within 18 months of making their claim, while in areas where the Pathways pilots were in operation this figure increased by 7.4% (Bewley et al, 2007). The impact on *existing* IB recipients is more difficult to gauge because they were not obliged to participate in the programme, but could do so voluntarily. Even if self-selection was not a source of bias, the effect size was very small, with the pilot areas adding just 0.7% to the return-to-work rate (Adam et al, 2008). Following roll-out of the Pathways initiative, its performance appears to be even more questionable. A recent white paper claims that although Pathways' initial performance had been encouraging, when the pilot was rolled out, no employment impact was found (DWP, 2009).

Despite limited effectiveness in returning long-term IB recipients to work, the Pathways approach lay at the heart of the government's strategy for returning a million IB recipients to work (DWP, 2008). A new work capability assessment (WCA) was implemented for all existing IB claimants, to assess their eligibility for the ESA that replaced IB; again, this sorted applicants according to their capacity for work, with the less impaired assigned to the work-related activity group and expected to prepare for return to work, while the more severely disabled receive a higher rate of benefit. Following Freud's (2007) recommendations, 'personalised back-to-work support' will be commissioned for all new and existing claimants of IB from private and voluntary sector providers, paid for by savings on benefits. The Fit for Work Service, which combines health and employment support, has run since April 2010 and will continue until at least March 2011; it is not clear if it will then stop in preparation for the Work Programme.

The South East Opportunities for Work (SEOW) initiative, which was independent of the government's Pathways initiative and funded by a local authority in south-east England, was among the first in the UK to provide a series of interventions designed specifically for supporting long-term IB recipients to return to employment. The aim was to enable 250 long-term (two years or more) IB recipients to return to employment for 13 weeks or more. The target was set in March 2005, with a completion date of March 2008, by which time it had returned 102 people to work (just over 40% of the target figure). The SEOW initiative launched in three areas, with high rates of long-term IB uptake, from June 2006 onwards. The names of the locations have been withheld to preserve anonymity, but they spanned the county from the suburbs of London to the south coast.

The programme involved private and not-for-profit providers as well as those in the public sector. Independent interventions were developed in the localities: *Area A (south coast)* adopted a vocational/training-based approach including employment-search and employment-related training; *Area B (mid-county town)* adopted a health-centred approach, comprising a condition management programme to improve physical and psychological fitness for work, including use of gym facilities, and vocational support provided in an afternoon Job Club; *Area C (outer London)* comprised two mobile support workers who provided services from a range of locations, including libraries, adult education centres and local cafes. The intervention included job-search and employment-related training. A fourth intervention was provided across the three localities. This ten-week programme was based on the theory of 'positive psychology' and aimed to promote resilience.

A team of university researchers was commissioned to evaluate the SEOW programme. This chapter is based on qualitative data collected as part of the evaluation. The aim is to arrive at a deeper understanding of how such initiatives address the reflexive reconstruction of self and social identity in order to inform future practice and policy development.

Methodology

Research design

The study aimed to access the lived experience of IB recipients, focusing on uptake of the SEOW interventions and how these experiences were invested with meaning. Qualitative methods are appropriate for in-depth exploration of meanings (Strauss and Corbin, 1998). Semi-structured interviews were used to get beneath the surface of informants' accounts and generate data that might not have been accessible using an alternative approach (Britten, 1995).

Selection and recruitment

Interviews were conducted with 12 informants between October and November 2007. Letters were sent to all registered service users (n = 100) by the local authority (to comply with data protection concerns).

Twenty-five replies were received. All respondents were telephoned a maximum of five times. If telephone contact could not be made, a follow-up letter was sent, inviting the potential participant to telephone the research team. All respondents completed a telephone interview in which the study was introduced, informed consent was sought and a short screening questionnaire was completed.

Three participants did not attend for interview and were unwilling to reschedule. A larger sample would be desirable, but long-term IB recipients are difficult to access and a lengthier approach to recruitment was not possible within the constraints of the study. Within the constraints imposed by the limited pool of service users willing to participate in the study, a maximum variation sampling strategy was used to select informants with a wide range of characteristics. Maximising the heterogeneity of the sample facilitated access to the broadest possible range of information, perspectives and experiences from a small number of participants. The strategy focused on achieving diversity in terms of age; gender; time on IB; reason for being on IB; and class (loosely defined as white- or blue-collar workers). Demographic data on all SEOW service users, or the wider population of IB recipients, is not available, so it is not possible to assess how typical the sample is. Table 8.1 shows the sample characteristics.

Data collection

The interviews were conducted by Rachel Black and Susan Kenyon in public buildings that were comfortable, quiet and afforded confidentiality. A topic guide was used to conduct semi-structured interviews lasting one to two hours. The topic guide covered reasons for incapacity; case history; experiences of seeking support; perceived obstacles to return to work; experiences of service uptake; satisfaction with services; suggestions for service improvements; expectations for the

Table 8.1: Sample characteristics

	A: South coast	B: Mid-county town	C: Outer London
Completed interviews	6	3	3
Age range	22-49	52-62	56-58
Gender (male:female)	3:3	3:0	3:0
Time on IB (years)	1-12	4-20	1-7
Reason on IB (physical:psychological:both)	2:0:4	2:1:0	1:1:1
Blue-collar:white-collar	2:4	2:1	2:1

future; and opportunities for informants to raise novel issues themselves. Interviews were recorded and transcribed by an agency.[1]

Findings

The experience of chronic pathology (physical, or psychosocial), coupled with long-term IB uptake, can damage selfhood and social identity.

The diminished self

Informants described how life on IB had diminished their sense of their own competence and resilience, often leading to a loss of agency in which they felt increasingly unable to cope with the demands of social engagement. Graham had been on IB for nine months at the time of interview due to a combination of epilepsy and alcohol problems, and describes how this has affected him:

> 'Because I'm not doing anything every day I'm starting to become a recluse.... you can sort of dig your own hole if you've got too much time on your hands ... you don't have to have a drink problem or get anxiety, but if you're not doing anything all day long things tend to well up in your mind ... I need to get back into work ... I don't feel great because I used to have a good job and everything else, but I wouldn't say I was positive right now.'

Graham describes the way in which social interaction strengthens the sense of selfhood by providing the individual with a sense of purpose. When social interaction is reduced, particularly through loss of employment, the web of meaning the individual has used to make sense of experience is also reduced, leaving the individual with a sense of 'anomie' or normlessness.

This diminished sense of selfhood can generate anxiety about the capacity to cope with return to work. In the following quotation, James, a senior manager on IB for six years following a nervous breakdown, describes his fear that the responsibilities of working life would prove too much for him:

> 'I don't mean the physical side of going back to work or anything like that ... I'm just petrified that someone's going

to put a bit of responsibility on me, and I don't ... I've had it. I don't need that.'

James's account illustrates how the diminished self entails a heightened sense of vulnerability. This is paradoxical. On the one hand, worklessness damages the self, but on the other hand, return to work may be experienced as a further threat to the self.

Uptake of mental health services can also have negative consequences for the self. Edward describes how being sectioned (involuntarily admitted to a mental institution under the terms of the 1983 Mental Health Act) further eroded his self-confidence and undermined his belief in his capacity to return to work:

'... my thought was to get better and to go back to work, before I was sectioned in 1988, which is a very traumatic experience and one that completely shattered whatever self-confidence I had. I thought I was just depressed and I could somehow cope with it, either with the help of psychotherapy and/or medication, but it was having the second breakdown and being sectioned which just broke ... I thought, I really have to be treated and that's all I could think about.'

Involuntary admission to a mental health institution may be necessary to protect the individual or others, but it is not surprising that it has consequences for the self, as it entails the suspension of the individual's right to govern their own activity, imposing a very potent label of incapacity that the individual is likely to reflect on and internalise. Other mental health interventions may be less dramatic, but by labelling the individual as mentally ill they may also affect selfhood and social identity. This is consistent with Goffman's analysis of the moral career of the mental patient, described in his classic work *Asylums* (Goffman, 1961).

The changes in selfhood brought about by long-term receipt of IB may also entail the adoption of a new way of presenting oneself to the world. This transformation of the self can be profound. In the following extract, Roger describes how his experience of being on IB for 13 years, coupled with a failed attempt to return to work, led him to construct an alternative set of beliefs about himself:

'I was just going, "Blow it, I'll be a kind of Bohemian nothing and just get drunk". I can try to romanticise what I was, my pathetic life I had, that was the only way to survive really, was to live this life and think of yourself as a photographer and artist who's living outside of society.'

This diminished sense of selfhood, therefore, has a dual dimension: it not only entails beliefs about the self, but also a way of presenting oneself to others; it becomes a way of managing one's social identity, in a way that is consistent with Giddens' (1991) work on the reflexive reconstruction of the self. This leads into the second theme.

Spoiled social identity

Having a biography that includes periods of illness and lengthy periods of worklessness has a profound effect on how one's identity is interpreted by others, especially potential employers. Interventions that focus on how to write a CV or how to dress for interview cannot fully disguise this damage to social identity. Moreover, as the theoretical accounts discussed above imply, there is a two-way relationship between selfhood and social identity: an IB recipient may present a social identity that emphasises their readiness for work, but if this identity is rejected by a potential employer, that rejection may well have consequences for the individual's sense of selfhood. The following quotation from John reveals how his biography, including drug addiction and time in prison, undermined both his social identity and his sense of selfhood:

> '… the drugs thing I was on for a long time, and came out of prison after that, just under a year, and I was ready to go clean healthy and all that. Not being able to get anything anywhere you slip again, don't you, you think everything's hopeless so you don't even try half the time, you think what's the point this will affect it, that will affect it, so you just you don't even try after a while, I mean I came here with no expectations.'

John's experiences have not only damaged his sense of self, but also how he believes his identity will be perceived by others. Return to work is not just about inner change to the self, but about reconstructing a plausible social identity, that is, demonstrating that one is a trustworthy, hardworking individual who will not cause problems for the employer. However, as the following quotation from Alice indicates, the reality of years out of work, coupled with ongoing impairment, have such a damaging impact on social identity that even those who are highly motivated to return to work struggle to persuade employers of their worth:

> 'I'd love to get back to work in any capacity. I really, really would love to get back to work but it's the flipping employers that say no ... I've got so much to offer. I've got a lot more than even some able-bodied people who really do not want to work ... but people just aren't interested; they just don't want to know.'

Ongoing health problems can affect the individual's ability to present a social identity that is likely to be attractive to potential employers. As Goffman's (1968) work on the relationship between stigma and identity predicts, even where ongoing pathology does not reduce the capacity for work, long-term IB recipients may still have to overcome the stigma associated with their previous problems. In this sense, labels of incapacity are 'sticky' and may continue to spoil the individual's social identity long after the initial problems have receded.

Relatively short bouts of illness and incapacity may have a correspondingly modest impact, but as the months and years pass by, incapacity for work becomes a more deeply entrenched aspect of the self and social identity. Edward, who had spent more than 20 years on IB, was aware of this difficulty:

> 'I think if you're out of work for a short time, then it's not such a big deal but the longer you're out and the longer you're ill the more difficult and the more remote the prospect of work becomes and it just becomes something that either is such a big step or one that just doesn't sound likely.'

Our evidence suggests that long-term uptake of IB can have a damaging effect on both the self and the social identity of the recipient that extends beyond that caused by the illness itself. It is this damage that many return-to-work interventions aim to address by actively reconstructing the self and social identity.

Reflexive reconstruction of self and social identity

Return-to-work initiatives strive to repair the damage to self and social identity that occurs during life on IB. This process of reconstruction is often non-linear. It is unlikely that IB recipients will *first* repair their sense of selfhood, *then* patch up their spoiled social identity, and *finally* return to work. More often, these stages are mutually dependent. Selfhood and social identity are mutually constitutive of each other – our sense of selfhood depends on interaction with others and their response to, and construction of, our social identity. Moreover, return to work often provides the essential context in which this process of reconstructing the self and social identity can occur. By returning to work and coping with its demands, the individual gains a strengthened sense of self-confidence and competence, while at the same time demonstrating their competence and reliability to others. Return to work is, therefore, an important part of the process of reconstructing the self and social identity, as the following quotation from Edward implies:

> '… part of the recovery process is to recover some sense of self and what I'm trying to do with my life. I know that I still want to find some way of finding an occupation while I still can and before it is too late for me, so I do want to get back to some sort of work, even if it is only initially stacking shelves in the local supermarket. I tried to explain to the occupational therapist that I do need to re-learn the whole process, the whole discipline of work.'

Return to work may bring benefits for the self and social identity, but making the return to work depends on the self and social identity being in pretty good shape to begin with. Edward describes this difficulty:

> '… the nature of the illness, certainly of the depression, is to withdraw, to do less and less, which is actually the last thing you should do. And the problem is, how to get somebody who's withdrawing, with less and less confidence, to do something … it doesn't make you very employable, so there are some inherent problems in how somebody like myself tries to cope with it, and also how other people get you somehow out of that state.'

Occasionally, employers may be willing to take on employees with a diminished sense of selfhood or a spoiled social identity, in recognition that work itself may enable them to overcome their difficulties and eventually fulfil their role effectively, particularly if the individual is a valued former employee seeking to return with the support of occupational health. However, many long-term IB recipients cannot rely on potential employers taking such an enlightened view and will find themselves competing against other applicants who pose less of a risk. It is often difficult, therefore, for long-term IB recipients to easily return to their previous career at an equivalent level of remuneration or status. For many, return to work often involves being prepared to accept low-paid, low-status jobs, or retraining to either increase their market value or to access careers with more job opportunities.

The need to embrace job change adds to the amount of work required in reconstructing the self and social identity. It is not just that long-term IB recipients need to repair damage to selfhood and social identity in order to return to their previous career; rather, they must actively reconstruct their self and social identity to fit with a new job. However, previous experiences of employment, prior to incapacity, often set in place a series of expectations, values and beliefs that were difficult to change, particularly for older informants who tended to have a relatively fixed idea of what constituted a suitable job for them. A key problem was status anxiety relating to the low pay or perceived low prestige of the jobs on offer. Brian described his reluctance to consider jobs that he felt lacked equivalent status to his previous work in the construction industry:

> '... they're going to go to me, "here's a job in this packing plant," do you understand what I mean, or, "here you are go sweep this road up," no, I ain't doing that. I'd much rather starve to death. I will do what work I want to do, yes. I've got a philosophy and I've taught my daughters it, if you ain't happy getting up and going to work in the morning, stay in your bed and jack your job in.'

This reluctance to take what were seen as inappropriate jobs points to an apparent paradox in the process of reconstructing the self and social identity. On one hand, informants displayed a diminished sense of selfhood, (lack of belief in their capacity to cope with work) and an awareness of their spoiled social identity (unattractiveness to potential employers), but on the other hand they also felt that the type of work they might be offered was beneath them. Although long-term IB recipients may have a diminished self and a spoiled identity, they are often not so diminished or spoilt that they are willing to take what they see as a low-status job. This places return-to-work interventions in a difficult position – on the one hand, trying to bolster the sense of selfhood and repair the social identity, but on the other hand lowering the individual's expectations of what they can aspire to. Later we will argue that a way out of this contradiction is to view return to work as a process in which taking a low-status job may be a brief stepping-stone. However, this process requires a highly individualised approach that is informed by a sound grasp of the individual's biography. Next we present evidence of the mismatch between the needs of informants and the interventions they were offered.

Mismatch between interventions and needs/wants of service users

The SEOW interventions comprised different combinations of coaching in job application skills, job search services, cognitive and behavioural therapy (CBT) and use of a gymnasium. The relatively fixed 'off-the-shelf' nature of the interventions meant that they could not be tailored to the diverse biographies of their users, resulting in a mismatch between what the interventions were offering and the specific needs and wants of the service users. Most users accessed the service by self-referral. There was little attempt to conduct a detailed needs assessment based on the individual's biography or circumstances and limited scope to vary the interventions to suit individual needs.

The interventions were insensitive to variations in the underlying physical/psycho/social pathology that had led to uptake of IB in the first place. Thus, some users complained that the interventions were not suitable for people whose pathology was as severe as their own; for example, Alice felt that the degree of physical disability resulting from her brain haemorrhage was not satisfactorily addressed:

> 'I'm sure they do an awful lot of good for people. I think this is just the wrong sort of thing for me, because I've got probably more needs ... I don't think this project is for seriously disabled people.'

The point is not that the interventions should have been widened to tackle different forms of physical, mental or social pathology (although they ought to have dovetailed with services that did), but rather that familiarity with the biographical information of the individuals concerned may have revealed that the interventions were inappropriate for them.

For others, the problem was that the interventions were not sensitive to other biographical factors, such as age, for example, Norman, a construction worker in his early 60s, described his frustration with a psychologist who was encouraging him to think 'outside the box' and consider alternative careers:

'... his idea of getting you back into work is to [encourage you to] come out of what he calls your comfort zone, where it could be ... like me, the only thing you've ever done in your life ... he turned round and said to me, "you've got to look outside the box," I said, "how can I look outside the box," I said, "I don't know nothing else." So I took five things (vacancies), he said, "try them," and they was all for factory work, warehouse work and all the rest of it. I thought, I can't do this. Anyway I phoned them all up for him and I put notes on the side of them, "no experience", "too old", and all the rest of it and I come back to him, I said, "there you are, outside the box."'

Several issues are apparent in the above extract: the deeply entrenched nature of previous occupational identities, the reluctance of older workers to respond positively to the invitation to change jobs, and the reluctance of employers to recruit under these circumstances. None of these factors is necessarily immutable, but again, greater awareness of the biography and circumstances of the individual would enable the likely effectiveness of this intervention to be assessed on a case-by-case basis.

Another commonly reported view was that the job search service and the training in job application skills were largely redundant, not just because other factors such as age or pathology made them unlikely to succeed, but because many informants felt that they already knew how to apply for jobs and could effectively search for work themselves. The following comment is from Alice:

'I just thought I'd be better off doing it on my own and using the internet access down at the library; going that way as opposed to being placed in jobs if you understand what I mean.... I end up telling them more than they're telling me and I know how to dress for an interview, thanks.'

The apparent mismatch between the needs and wants of the service users and what the interventions delivered may have contributed to the limited effectiveness of the SEOW programme, but more than that, there was a sense from some informants that their involvement with the programme had caused them disappointment and distress. Again, Alice comments:

> 'No, it definitely made me feel so low. I was quite emotional at the time and it made me feel worse…. I don't mind going through the rigmarole, but the whole thing, you know, being told we'll be in touch or whatever and having my time wasted. I don't give up easily on anything but, you know, bit soul destroying, yes bit soul destroying. That's why I was upset before.'

It is unsurprising that when individuals participate in a return-to-work programme and emerge without a job that they do not view the experience as a positive one, but this is particularly acute if the interventions reinforce the individual's sense of hopelessness, or the belief that nothing can be done to improve their circumstances.

In short, the evidence suggests that there was a mismatch between what the interventions were offering and what the users needed or wanted. The interventions were based on the assumption that barriers to return to work were mainly to do with lack of job search skills or motivational issues that could be addressed by CBT or gym membership. Very rarely did this match with expressed needs or preferences; thus, although many informants felt that SEOW was worthwhile for unspecified others, most felt that it was not appropriate for them.

Discussion

Theoretical framework

Figure 8.1 illustrates the theoretical framework derived from the analysis. The top of the diagram shows the physical, and psychosocial pathologies that can lead to uptake of IB. Life on IB can lead to a diminished sense of selfhood and a spoiled social identity. Return to work requires not just the reconstruction of the self and social identity, but also the development of strategies for the successful presentation of the self, particularly to potential employers. A double-headed arrow indicates the reciprocal relationship between self and social identity. There is a feedback loop between uptake of employment opportunities and the reconstruction of self and social identity.

The SEOW interventions map on to the framework at three points. CBT and use of the gym both addressed the problem of the diminished self; aiming to build a heightened sense of competence, resilience and openness to job change. Training in job application skills addressed the presentation of the self, aiming to enable individuals to manage how they would be perceived by potential employers. Finally, the job search

Figure 8.1: Theoretical framework

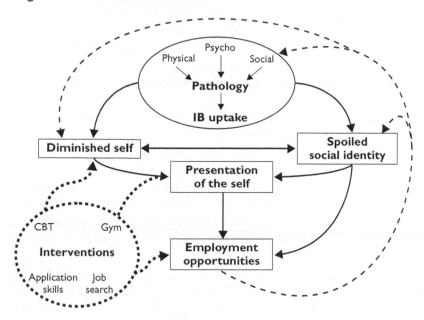

service aimed to identify employment opportunities and to encourage individuals to consider a wider range of jobs. Having briefly outlined the framework, we now examine its components more closely.

Self and social identity

Self and social identity relate to the project of returning IB recipients to work in a number of ways. The self is the repository of our motivations and our beliefs about our capabilities, skills and resilience – it includes the knowledge we refer to when answering questions such as 'Am I able to return to work?' or 'Am I able or willing to do that type of work?' Scrutiny of an applicant's social identity is the means by which potential employers decide whether to employ someone – it includes the knowledge that others refer to in order to answer questions such as 'Will this person be able to do the job?', 'Will they be reliable and hardworking?', 'Are they likely to take sick leave?'.

Long-term uptake of IB can do substantial damage to both the self and social identity, which reduces the likelihood of an individual returning to work; after a year on IB, recipients are more likely to die or retire on IB than they are to return to work (Waddell and Aylward, 2005). For this reason, many return-to-work interventions attempt to repair this damage to the self. To use Giddens' (1991) terminology (which, of course, such interventions never do), the aim of such initiatives is to support the reflexive reconstruction of self and social identity. The question is, why have such interventions had only limited success and what can be done to make them more effective?

Lessons for policy and the development of effective interventions

Our findings provide a rich description of the experiences of long-term IB recipients as they engage with interventions designed to return them to work. What emerges is paradoxical; informants reported *common* problems of damage to their sense of selfhood and to their social identity, but these problems were grounded in *individual* experiences and biography. This paradox poses a problem because although the desired outcomes are broadly similar, interventions that are insensitive to variations in experience and biography are likely to be irrelevant, ineffective or possibly even harmful.

Interventions that aim to find job opportunities, improve the formatting of the individual's CV or develop interview skills are not appropriate for those who are already competent in these skills or who have such damage to their selfhood or social identity that they are unlikely to be effective. Similarly, psychological interventions may be inappropriate for people with problems that are essentially physical or social. The inappropriate use of such interventions is not only ineffective, but may also further harm the individual's sense of selfhood, first, by raising expectations that will not be met, and second, by reinforcing a diminished sense of selfhood, leading individuals to conclude that because such an intervention has been prescribed they *must* be in need of it. What is required is a much more individualised approach to case management that assesses an individual's specific needs and coordinates a series of highly appropriate interventions to address them.

Recent policy statements (DWP, 2008, 2009) including the 2011 Welfare Reform Bill recognise the need for personalised care, but the mechanism for service delivery might militate against this. The Freud report (2007) proposes a pluralistic model in which providers from public, private and voluntary organisations bid to provide services that will be funded from savings on benefits generated by IB recipients returning to work for at least 13 weeks. The Work Programme, which the government aims to introduce in summer 2011, follows this pluralism (DWP, 2010). The danger is that private sector providers in particular may adopt 'off-the-shelf' interventions that may coerce IB recipients into accepting inappropriate work that is sustained for only a short time after the 13-week target. It is possible to envisage a scenario in which individuals are harmed by this process, leading to a 'revolving door' of relatively short-term episodes of employment and return to benefit uptake. Current details available regarding the Work Programme suggest that providers can earn an extra sustainment fee by keeping someone in work for only four weeks (DWP, 2010b).

The pluralistic model of service delivery may also hamper coordination of different interventions. The National Audit Office (NAO, 2010) recently reported on the effectiveness of Pathways. This report found that Jobcentre Plus Pathways performed better than provider-led Pathways in supporting claimants into employment. The report suggested that provider-led contractors probably underestimated the complex needs of Pathways claimants. Such problems are not insurmountable, but services will need to be commissioned carefully if such pitfalls are to be avoided.

Our findings also support the need for a broader shift in workplace initiatives to facilitate return to work. Partly this would entail initiatives and incentives designed to change employers' attitudes towards the employment of people whose social identity has been spoiled by long-term uptake of IB. This is particularly pressing for individuals whose uptake of IB is linked with psychological or mental health problems and Dame Carol Black's (2008) ongoing review of employment and mental health provides an important opportunity to address this issue. Our findings suggest that there are IB recipients whose needs are such that some form of sheltered employment, organised or commissioned by government, may be required either as an alternative to, or stepping-stone towards, regular mainstream employment. This approach has been used widely in the US and a recent review of randomised controlled trials suggests that supported employment programmes (in which clients are placed in employment and receive on the job support) are more effective than pre-vocational interventions in returning mentally ill clients to work (Crowther et al, 2001). Supported employment programmes have also proven effective in returning patients with traumatic brain injuries to work, although success is dependent on the characteristics of the client (Wehman et al, 1993). Such provision also requires careful planning to ensure that individuals are not ghettoised or further stigmatised. The most up-to-date Work Programme prospectus, of November 2010, does not directly address employer attitudes, although there is latitude for providers to manage employers however they see fit (DWP, 2010).

The government's proposals for IB reform offer an opportunity for improving the lives of individuals who have previously been largely neglected by public policy. Our findings support much of what is proposed, but they also suggest that progress towards the target of returning one million IB recipients to paid employment will depend on the commissioning of interventions that are highly sensitive to the individual biographies, circumstances and needs of the IB recipient. The Work Programme emphasises that providers will be given 'the flexibility to design support based on customer need' (DWP, 2010, p 2) and recognises the 'failings of previous employment services which were inflexible, short term and failed to support the hardest to reach customers' (DWP, 2010, p 2). Listening to the voices of IB recipients will be an important aspect of service development and whatever form they take, interventions will need to be rigorously evaluated. Qualitative research has limitations in terms of representativeness and transferability, particularly when informants come from a vulnerable group that is difficult to access, so our findings should be treated with a degree of circumspection. However, qualitative studies of this kind can provide policymakers and service providers with an in-depth understanding of how users experience service uptake and how interventions affect their sense of selfhood and social identity. These factors are likely to play an important role in sustained return to work and should be included in any evaluation alongside quantitative measures of the numbers leaving benefit.

Note

[1] For data analysis, a twofold analytical strategy was adopted in order first to preserve the individual illness narratives of informants in order to reveal how the experience of IB uptake varies across the life-course and in response to personal circumstances (Greenhalgh and Hurwitz, 1999; Bury, 2001) and second, to identify common themes by 'breaking the data' and reorganising them under thematic headings. The first part of the analytical strategy was achieved by focusing on individual transcripts and producing descriptive summaries of each informant's 'story' or narrative, while the second was achieved by using a thematic content analysis method (Green and Thorogood, 2004), informed by some of the techniques of grounded theory (Strauss, 1987). Atlas.ti software was used to manage the analytical process. An iterative approach was adopted, beginning with open coding of each transcript, followed by a process of recoding in which codes were compared and modified as the analysis developed. Relationships between codes were explored and combined into themes, which in turn were used to develop a theoretical framework (see Figure 8.1).

With respect to research ethics, approval for the study was granted by the local authority's Research Ethics Committee. Informed consent was obtained from all participants. In order to protect anonymity, quotations are presented with minimal descriptors, some biographical details have been disguised and pseudonyms have been used throughout.

Further reading

DWP (Department for Work and Pensions) (2010) 'The Work Programme prospectus – November 2010', www.dwp.gov.uk/docs/work-prog-prospectus-v2.pdf

Goffman, E. (1968) *Stigma notes on the management of spoiled identity*, Harmondsworth: Penguin.

NAO (National Audit Office) (2010) *Support to incapacity benefits claimants through Pathways to Work*, Report HC21, London: Her Majesty's Stationery Office.

Waddell, G. and Aylward, M. (2005) *The scientific and conceptual basis of incapacity benefits*, London: The Stationery Office.

Wainwright, D. (2008) 'Illness behaviour and the discourse of health', in D. Wainwright (ed) *A sociology of health*, London: Sage Publications, pp 76-96.

References

Abramson, L.Y., Seligman, M.E.P. and Teasdale, J.D. (1978) 'Learned helplessness in humans: critique and reformulation', *Journal of Abnormal Psychology*, vol 87, pp 49-74.

Adam, S., Bozio, A., Emmerson, C., Greenberg, D. and Knight, G. (2008) *A cost-benefit analysis of Pathways to Work for new and repeat incapacity benefits claimants*, DWP Research Report No 498, London: Her Majesty's Stationery Office.

Avineri, S. (1968) *The social and political thought of Karl Marx*, Cambridge: Cambridge University Press.

Ball, D. (1972) 'Self and identity in the context of deviance: the case of criminal abortion', in R.A. Scot and J.D. Douglas (eds) *Theoretical perspectives on deviance*, New York, NY: Basic Books.

Bambra, C.I. (2008) 'Incapacity benefit reform and the politics of ill health', *British Medical Journal*, vol 337, p 1452.

Bandura, A. (1977) 'Self-efficacy: toward a unifying theory of behavioural change', *Psychological Review*, vol 84, pp 191-215.

Bandura, A. (1991) 'Self-efficacy mechanism in physiological activation and health-promoting behavior', in J.I.V. Madden (ed) *Neurobiology of learning, emotion and affect*, New York, NY: Raven, pp 229-69.

Becker, H. (1973) *Outsiders: Studies in the sociology of deviance* (2nd edn), New York, NY: Free Press.

Bewley, H., Dorsett, R. and Haile, G. (2007) *The impact of Pathways to Work*, DWP Research Report No 435, London: Her Majesty's Stationery Office.

Black, C. (2008) *Working for a healthier tomorrow*, London: The Stationery Office.

Britten, N. (1995) 'Qualitative research: qualitative interviews in medical research', *British Medical Journal*, vol 311, pp 251-3.

Burke, P. (1980) 'The self: measurement requirements from an interactionist perspective', *Social Psychology Quarterly*, vol 43, pp 18-29.

Bury, M. (2001) 'Illness narratives, fact or fiction?', *Sociology of Health and Illness*, vol 23, no 1, pp 263-85.

Cooley, C. (1981) 'Self as sentiment and reflection', in G. Stone and H. Faberman (eds) *Social psychology through symbolic interactionism*, New York, NY: Wiley.

Crowther, R.E., Marshall, M., Bond, G.R. and Huxley, P. (2001) 'Helping people with severe mental illness to obtain work: systematic review', *British Medical Journal*, vol 322, no 7280, p 204.

DWP (Department for Work and Pensions) (2006) *A new deal for welfare: Empowering people to work*, Cm 6730, London: The Stationery Office.

DWP (2008) *Raising expectations and increasing support: Reforming welfare for the future,* Cm 7506, London: The Stationery Office.

DWP (2009) *Building Britain's recovery: Achieving full employment*, Cm 7751, London: The Stationery Office.

DWP (2010a) 'The Work Programme prospectus – November 2010', www.dwp.gov.uk/docs/work-prog-prospectus-v2.pdf

DWP (2010b) 'Draft: Call-off terms and conditions for the Work Programme', www.dwp.gov.uk/docs/work-prog-draft-terms.pdf

Douglas, J. (1984) 'The emergence, security and growth of the sense of self', in J. Kortaba and A. Fontana (eds) *The existential self in society*, Chicago, IL: University of Chicago Press.

Fideler, P.A. (2005) *Social welfare in pre-industrial England: The old Poor Law tradition (Social History in Perspective)*, London: Palgrave Macmillan.

Field, D. (1974) 'Introduction', in D. Field (ed) *Social psychology for sociologists*, London: Nelson.

Field, F. (2007) 'Less carrot, more stick', *Daily Telegraph*, www.telegraph. co.uk/opinion/main.jhtml?xml=/opinion/2007/03/06/do0602.xml, accessed 31 July 2009.

Freud, D. (2007) *Reducing dependency, increasing opportunity: Options for the future of welfare to work*, Independent report to the Department for Work and Pensions, Leeds: Corporate Document Services.

Gergen, K. (1971) *The concept of self*, New York, NY: Holt, Rinehart and Winston.

Giddens, A. (1991) *Modernity and self-identity: Self and society in the late modern age,* Cambridge: Polity Press.

Goffman, E. (1968) *Stigma: Notes on the management of spoiled identity,* Harmondsworth: Penguin.

Goffman, E. (1961) *Asylums: Essays on the social situation of mental patients and other inmates,* Harmondsworth: Penguin.

Green, J. and Thorogood, N. (2004) *Qualitative methods for health research,* London: Sage Publications.

Greenhalgh, T. and Hurwitz, B. (1999) 'Why study narrative?', *British Medical Journal,* vol 318, no 7175, pp 48-50.

Grint, K. (2005) *The sociology of work* (5th edn), Cambridge: Polity Press.

Heath, A. (1976) *Rational choice and social exchange,* Cambridge: Cambridge University Press.

James, W. (1892) *Psychology: The briefer course,* New York, NY: Holt, Rinehart and Winston.

Katz, M. (1989) *The undeserving poor: From the war on poverty to the war on welfare,* New York, NY: Pantheon Books.

Lazarus, R.S. and Folkman, S. (1984) 'Coping and adaptation', in W.D. Gentry (ed) *The handbook of behavioral medicine,* New York, NY: Guilford, pp 282-325.

Leonard, N.H., Beauvais, L.L. and Scholl, R.W. (1999) 'Work motivation: the incorporation of self-concept based processes', *Human Relations,* vol 52, no 8, pp 969-98.

McCall, G. and Simmons, J. (1966) *Identities and interactions,* New York, NY: Free Press, p 70.

Mead, G.H. (1934) *Mind, self and society: From the standpoint of the social behaviourist,* Chicago, IL: University of Chicago Press.

Mead, G.H. (1981) 'Self as social object', in G. Stone and H. Faberman (eds) *Social psychology through symbolic interactionism,* New York, NY: Wiley.

Mechanic, D. (1999) 'Sociological dimensions of illness behavior', *Social Science and Medicine,* vol 41, no 9, pp 1207-16.

NAO (National Audit Office) (2010) *Support to incapacity benefits claimants through Pathways to Work,* Report HC 21, London: The Stationery Office.

Page, L.A. and Wessely, S. (2003) 'Medically unexplained symptoms: exacerbating factors in the doctor-patient encounter', *Journal of the Royal Society of Medicine,* vol 96, no 5, pp 223-7.

Rotter, J.B. (1975) 'Some problems and misconceptions related to the construct of internal versus external control of reinforcement', *Journal of Consulting and Clinical Psychology*, vol 43, no 1, pp 56-67.

Strauss, A. (1987) *Qualitative analysis for social scientists*, Cambridge: Cambridge University Press.

Strauss, A. and Corbin, J. (1998) *Basics of qualitative research*, Thousand Oaks, CA: Sage Publications.

Twaddle, A. (1973) 'Illness and deviance', *Social Science and Medicine*, vol 7, pp 751-62.

Waddell, G. and Aylward, M. (2005) *The scientific and conceptual basis of incapacity benefits*, London: The Stationery Office.

Waddell, G. and Burton, A.K. (2004) *Concepts of rehabilitation for the management of common health problems*, London: The Stationery Office.

Wagner, H.R. (1970) 'Introduction', in A. Shutz (ed) *On phenomenology and social relations*, Chicago, IL: University of Chicago Press.

Wainwright, D. (2004) 'The benefits of incapacity', in M. O'Donnell (ed) *Beyond understanding: Getting to the root causes of ill health*, Chief Medical Officer's Report, Dorking: Unum Provident, www.unum.co.uk/NR/rdonlyres/85881581-D365-4C15-8772-D46BF24C6CF3/0/CMOReport2004.pdf , accessed 31 July 2009.

Wainwright, D. (2008) 'Illness behaviour and the discourse of health', in D. Wainwright (ed) *A sociology of health*, London: Sage Publications, pp 76-96.

Wehman, P., Kregel, J., Sherron, P., Nguyen, S., Kreutzer, J., Fry, R. and Zasler, N. (1993) 'Critical factors associated with the successful supported employment placement of patients with severe traumatic brain injury', *Brain Injury*, vol 7, no 1, pp 31-44.

Weinstein, E. and Deutschberger, P. (1963) 'Some dimensions of altercasting', *Sociometry*, vol 26, pp 355-60.

Young, J.T. (2004) 'Illness behaviour: a selective review and synthesis', *Sociology of Health & Illness*, vol 26, no 1, pp 1-31.

NINE

The fall of work stress and the rise of wellbeing

David Wainwright and Michael Calnan

Introduction

Over the past 30 years, the discourse of work stress has become one of the key frames of reference by which people make sense of the problems they encounter in their working lives (Wainwright and Calnan, 2002). In 2007/08, the UK Labour Force Survey found that 17% of workers reported that their job was very or extremely stressful; a third had discussed work stress with their line manager; 442,000 workers felt that stress was making them ill; and work stress accounted for 13.5 million lost working days (ONS, 2009). As well as charting the extent of the 'epidemic', this self-reported data also reveal that notions of work stress have moved from the sphere of academic debate into the public domain, providing a web of meaning through which workers can make sense of their experiences at work.

The discourse of work stress may be on everyone's lips, but we wish to argue that it is about to fall. The academic theories of work stress that underpin the popular discourse are riven with conceptual problems and methodological difficulties, and policymakers and employers are increasingly turning to the currently rather amorphous concept of 'wellbeing' to provide an alternative means of understanding and addressing the relationship between work and health. The aim of this chapter is to elucidate the fall of work stress and the rise of wellbeing, and to argue for a conception of wellbeing that is theoretically grounded in the social determinants of illness behaviour and resilience.

The popular discourse of work stress

During the second half of the 20th century, ideas about work stress crossed the boundary between science and popular discourse. Today these notions are so deeply embedded in the popular imagination that they appear naturalised and universal, so much so that it is difficult to imagine a time before work stress, or a place where it might not be found. In this sense, we can speak of a popular discourse of work stress – a set of shared assumptions, norms, expectations and ways of being in the world that collectively provide a web of meaning through which adverse experiences at work can be interpreted and made sense of. In our book on the making of the work stress epidemic, we charted the broad contours of this popular discourse by analysing accounts of work stress that appeared in the print media, in grey literature produced by trade unions, government agencies and other organisations, and in qualitative interviews we had conducted with people suffering from work stress (Wainwright and Calnan, 2002). The results of this analysis are represented in Figure 9.1.

The top three boxes in the diagram describe the cause-and-effect relationship that is widely held to account for the rise of the work stress epidemic. Changes in work, including the intensification of production, greater job insecurity and longer working hours, are deemed to have given rise to widespread and grossly increased feelings of psychological distress and strain or pressure. The fight-or-flight response is often invoked to describe the physiological processes that

Figure 9.1:The popular discourse of work stress

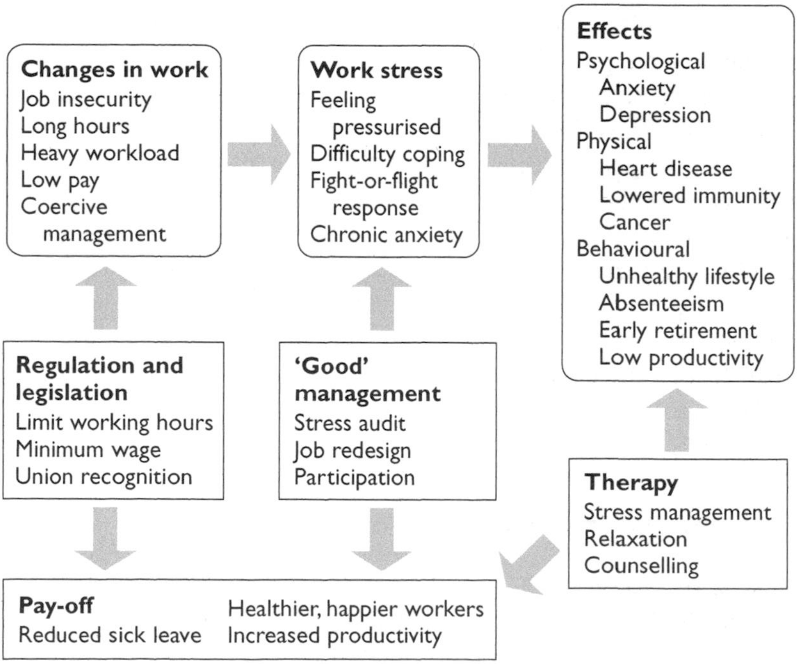

Source: Adapted from Wainwright and Calnan (2002)

underpin this response, often framed within a rhetoric drawn from evolutionary psychology that claims that this adaptive mechanism, evolved to help our ancestors deal with the acute threats they faced as hunter-gatherers, has become dysfunctional because the threats faced in the modern workplace are so constant that the worker's hypothalamic-pituitary-adrenal axis is in a chronic state of arousal. Chronic stress is perceived to cause a very wide range of psychological, physical and behavioural pathologies, including clinical anxiety and depression, heart disease, lowered immunity and even some cancers, as well as increasing rates of smoking, alcohol consumption and poor diet, and prompting absenteeism, early retirement and diminished productivity.

The putative solutions to the work stress epidemic broadly align with this three-stage model of cause and effect. Thus, adverse changes in work are to be tackled by regulation and legislation to limit the length of the working week, establish a minimum wage and recognise the role of unions in protecting the interests of workers (some of these measures have been introduced in the UK since the election of a Labour government in 1997). At the organisational level, job strain is to be tackled by 'good' management. This usually entails conducting a stress audit to identify those workers most at risk and developing a number of organisational changes, including job redesign and worker participation, to ease the pressure. Finally, at the level of the individual, numerous therapeutic solutions are posited to ameliorate the effects of stress, including the adoption of stress management techniques, counselling sessions and various methods to induce relaxation, such as massage and meditation.

Many of the proposals for tackling the work stress epidemic entail significant costs for employers, yet the pay-off for introducing them is widely perceived to be not just a happier healthier workforce, but also a dramatic reduction in sick leave and increased productivity. The implication is that everyone will benefit from the proposed measures.

Beguiling though the popular discourse of work stress may be, it is our contention that it is based on a conceptually flawed notion of the relationship between paid employment and health. We begin our critique by addressing the first question that sociologists should ask of any new social phenomenon – why now?

Answering the 'Why now?' question

As Figure 9.1 implies, the popular discourse of work stress provides its own explanation of why work stress came to prominence as a public issue from the late 1970s onwards. Central to this explanation is the end of the post-war boom, which, at least in the UK context, is usually dated in the mid-1970s when the Organization of the Petroleum Exporting Countries/International Monetary Fund crisis sparked recession and a restructuring of the relationship between labour and capital. The crisis hastened the decline of manufacturing and extractive industries and led to the election of a Conservative government in 1979, led by Margaret Thatcher and committed to the curtailment of trade union rights, privatisation of nationalised industries and public utilities, and cuts to public services and welfare spending.

These broad economic and political changes are often claimed to have brought about a rapid transformation in the nature of work, including greater job insecurity or 'the end of a job for life'; an increase in the number of hours worked per week or 'the long hours culture'; the intensification of work or 'the return to the sweat-shop', and a reduction in the amount of time spent with family and friends or 'poor work–life balance'. The assumption is that working life has become far more onerous than it was for earlier generations and that for many workers the psychological strain of modern working life has passed the limit of human physical and mental endurance, leading not just to high levels of work stress but also to serious psychological and physical harm.

The claim that the work stress epidemic is solely a response to a rapid and substantial decline in the quality of working life roughly during the decade after 1975 has an intuitive appeal and it is easy to find exemplars of corporate downsizing, coercive management techniques and loss of work-related rights and privileges (Burke and Cooper, 2000). The difficulty arises when we try to move from individual case studies and anecdotes to rigorous empirical evidence of broad changes in the quality and demands of working life. The field is riven with methodological difficulties and has provided fertile ground for academic debate, of which the economist Francis Green has provided a comprehensive and even-handed review (Green, 2006). Two key problems are the reliance on self-report data and the tendency for averages (for the workforce as a whole) to mask polarisation between different groups of workers.

Self-report data on appraisals of changes in working life are questionable because they rely on a subjective assessment rather than an objective measurement of changes, for example, workers might be asked, 'Do you feel that you are working harder now than you were 12 months ago?'. This appraisal could be shaped by several factors apart from an actual intensification of work; not least, the discourse of work stress is so deeply embedded in the popular imagination that it may itself play a role in shaping perceptions of working conditions.

The aggregation of data to reveal average changes in work across the whole workforce is problematic because it inevitably masks wide variations between groups. Disaggregating the data leads to the rather banal conclusion that work has improved for some workers while getting worse for others.

Setting aside methodological difficulties, what can confidently be concluded about changes in the nature of work that occurred from the mid-1970s through the 1980s? Green's (2006) analysis reveals a mixed and complicated picture. If we take job tenure (the amount of time spent in a particular job) and job insecurity, the evidence is quite surprising. The perception is that there are 'no more jobs for life', that globalisation and increased competition have forced employers to hire and fire at will in response to market fluctuations. This uncertainty about future employment is often mooted as a major cause of anxiety and stress for modern workers, but is it real? Data from the United States suggest that the proportion of workers who were highly insecure regarding the risk of job loss, remained at around 11% (plus or minus 3%) from 1977, (Bureau of Labour Statistics, cited in Green, 2006, p 135). Data for the UK only go back to 1986, but again the number of workers rating the likelihood of job loss at evens, quite likely, or very likely, fell from around 16% in 1986 and 1997 to 12% in 2001 (Social Change and Economic Life Initiative, cited in Green, 2006, p 133). These aggregated data may well mask a redistribution of insecurity between different groups of workers. For instance, Green notes that in the UK professional workers and those in the financial sector in particular may have become particularly insecure in the mid-1990s, (perhaps even more so in 2008-09). Even so, Green (2006, p 147) concludes that '... it is not accurate to describe work in the modern industrialised world as especially insecure ... one cannot scientifically sustain proclamations of a *secular* upward shift in insecurity' (emphasis in original).

Green finds greater evidence to support the claim that work became more intense during the 1980s and 1990s, at least in the UK context. For example, in 1986, workers were asked to compare their current job with the one they had five years before; 38% said that their work speed had increased and 56% claimed their work required more effort (Green, 2006, p 51). The Workplace Industrial Relations Survey posed a similar question in 1990, asking workers' representatives to compare the current work effort in their establishment with that of three years earlier. Among establishments characterised by manual work, 26% reported that work effort was a little higher and 30% a lot higher. For non-manual establishments, the percentages were 22 and 46 respectively (Green, 2006, p 52). Across the 1990s, a similar pattern emerges: in 1992,

32% of workers surveyed strongly agreed that their job required hard work and by 2001 this had risen to 38% (Green, 2006, p 55). Although the evidence is less compelling, Green finds a similar pattern in most European Union countries and in the US and Canada.

If workers feel that their work effort has increased, what does this actually signify? Is this perception an unmediated reflection of an objective increase in effort, or does it stem from other factors? For example, when workers compared their current work intensity with that of three or four years earlier, might their recollections have been coloured by the social desirability of claiming an increase, or by immersion in a broader cultural narrative that emphasised the deleterious effects of capitalist globalisation? These questions cannot be answered using the data sets that inform Green's analysis.

Easier to test are the assertions that Britain has developed a 'long hours culture' in which individuals are spending more time at work and thereby upsetting their work–life balance. Rather than relying on workers' subjective assessments of whether they are working longer hours than in the past, there are reliable and objective international data on the average annual hours actually worked per employed person. Comparing the hours worked in 1979, 1983, 1990 and 2003, it becomes apparent that for many countries, including Belgium, Finland, France, Germany, Italy, Korea, Japan and Norway, average weekly working hours fell from the early 1980s. Other countries – the UK, United States, Greece, Sweden, Canada and Australia – experienced little change, and a marked increase in the length of the working week cannot be found in any industrialised country (Green, 2006, p 45).

In summary, there is little evidence to support the claim that contemporary work is *generally* less secure than it was in the 1970s, or that the average working week has increased since then. There is some evidence to suggest an intensification of work effort over this period, although much of this intensification is not the result of coercive management forcing workers to work harder for the same or lower wages. Indeed, many countries, including the UK, that show an increase in work effort have also enjoyed substantial wage increases over the same period, and much of the incentive to work harder is driven by the worker's desire to increase earnings (Green, 2006).

Even if we accept the notion that work has become harder since the mid-1970s, at least for some groups within the workforce, consideration of changes over a longer time period reveals that even in this worst-case scenario the pattern is one of substantial and protracted improvements in working life, followed by the most marginal reversals. Take the length of the working week. In the 1860s, London's fitters and turners worked nearly 60 hours per week, virtually every week of the year. By 1968 manual workers had two to three weeks' paid leave per year and the average working week had fallen to 40 hours. A similar pattern exists for all groups of workers for whom reliable data are available (Green, 2001).

Long-term changes in the intensity of work and the psychological demands placed on the worker are harder to gauge, but it is difficult to imagine that life as a coal miner before the industry was nationalised, or as a docker before the National Dock Labour Scheme was introduced, could have been any less arduous than employment in, say, a modern call-centre. Indeed, factory work in the late 19th century (and well into the 20th) was often characterised by direct and brutal coercion by an overseer, constant uncertainty about staying in work, and very little in the way of a welfare safety net (Hobsbawm, 1968).

Yet prior to the 1970s, the discourse of work stress barely existed outside of academia and there is no evidence of a work stress epidemic before this time. It might be argued that work stress existed in these times but went undetected because science lacked the concepts or the methods to reveal it. However, it is difficult to believe that in the golden age of British epidemiology in the immediate post-war period, men like Townsend, Abel-Smith, Boyd Orr, Morris, Titmuss and others, so adept at unearthing evidence of the health effects of tobacco, poverty, unemployment and exercise, could miss a phenomenon as putatively widespread as work stress (see Davey Smith et al, 2001 for an overview of the achievements of this generation of social epidemiologists).

In summary, it is difficult to sustain the claim that the work stress epidemic is an unmediated response to the physical or psychological demands of modern employment. Work may have become worse since 1975 for some sectors of the workforce, but even if this is so, it is hard to believe that the demands placed on them are so intense that some natural 'breaking point' has been surpassed that inevitably leads to a high incidence of mental and physical morbidity. The failure of the discourse of work stress to arrive at a persuasive explanation of why the phenomenon arose is a fundamental weakness of the paradigm. We now turn to a closer consideration of the conceptual limitations of work stress.

Limitations of the concept of work stress

The concept of stress is derived from physics and engineering, where it is used to describe the application of force to an inanimate object or structure; imagine a metal bar bending under the pressure of weights, or a road bridge buckling under the strain of traffic. In this sense, stress offers a powerful *metaphor* for mental health, providing an insight into the human psyche suffering under the burden of social pressures. The problem is that stress has become a dead metaphor; that is, we no longer think that mental health problems are *like* the notion of stress in engineering, rather we assume that stress *is* the process by which mental health is impaired. This is essentially the error of positivism – the assumption that human behaviour can be understood using the same methodological and conceptual apparatus that the natural sciences have applied to the natural world. The problem is that such an approach is literally mechanistic and overlooks the role of consciousness in mediating the relationship between lived experience and its impact on the individual and their subsequent behaviour. Thus, an inanimate object like a road bridge *does* have an objectively measurable and fixed breaking point in terms of the weight and volume of traffic that will lead to its failure. It does not matter what the bridge 'thinks' about the threat posed by the traffic, or about its own capacity to 'cope', or about what others will think of it if it fails. Yet these thoughts and appraisals are fundamental in determining how humans respond to the challenges and demands they encounter in their daily lives (Lazarus and Folkman, 1984).

Changes in the intensity or duration of work do not affect the individual in the same way that a heavy lorry affects a buckling bridge. Individuals interpret and make sense of these changes; they reflect on their capacity to cope with the change and consider the different ways in which they might respond. This process of appraisal is inherently social, that is, it depends on interaction with other members of the social network, both at work and at home, as well as on broader cultural norms and expectations about reasonable levels of workload or appropriate responses to change. The response is also shaped by prevailing structural and institutional arrangements. Thus one of the reasons there was no work stress epidemic prior to the 1970s, despite the prevalence of hardship at work, may have been due to the existence of effective trade unions that offered an alternative strategy for interpreting and responding to negative experiences at work.

Recognising the social nature of appraisal leads into a further criticism of the work stress model – the extent to which it offers a broadly mono-causal account of mental health and illness behaviour by focusing exclusively on the role of work characteristics as the cause of stress and its various psychological and physical correlates. Despite an ongoing fascination with biology, modern psychiatry largely eschews mono-causal theories of emotional states and mental health status (Paris, 2010). Our mental life, it seems, is always multicausal, stemming from a complex interaction of genetic inheritance, upbringing, education and interaction with a broad web of significant others. Experiences at work may clearly play a role, perhaps even a fundamental role, but they cannot plausibly be posited as the *only* cause of psychiatric distress. Even when individuals declare problems at work to be the sole cause of their distress, it is worth pausing to consider how they came to construct this account of their problems, and to recognise that the popular discourse of work stress, as a potent cultural force, may itself play a role in such attributions. The way in which the discourse of work stress posits particular causes of emotional problems at work, and its prescriptions about how they should be tackled, may appear inherently neutral, but in essence may reflect (and reproduce) marginalisation of the experiences of particular groups, for example women (Meyerson, 1998).

While the discourse of work stress can be criticised for excluding non-work-related factors from the aetiology of psychiatric distress, ironically it can also be criticised for its lack of specificity. Thus, virtually any negative job characteristic can be cited as a cause of stress, from heavy workload to background noise, too many emails or unsatisfactory furniture. This wide range of factors is claimed to affect a large number of emotional states, classically the fight-or-flight response, but also anxiety, depression, anger or despair. Finally, these negative emotions are often linked to a very wide range of mental and physical pathologies, including burnout, clinical depression, coronary heart disease, lowered immune function and even some cancers. What is really being claimed is that almost any adverse experience at work can give rise to almost any negative emotion, which in turn can give rise to an exceptionally wide range of illnesses. This lack of specificity makes for very poor epidemiology.

The strongest evidence for the theory of work stress has been produced by epidemiologists who have attempted to be more specific about both the job characteristics that cause stress and the health problems that exposure to these 'stressors' gives rise to, for example coronary heart disease (CHD); see Stansfeld and Marmot (2002) for a review of the evidence base. CHD is a clearly defined and measurable outcome, and researchers have attempted to define equally clear job strain variables. Two models are particularly prominent in the literature, the demands-control-support (DCS) model, which predicts that job strain will occur when working conditions make heavy demands on the worker, but provide low levels of control over how the work is done, and little in the way of social support from managers and colleagues (Karasek and Theorell, 1990). A second approach, the effort-reward-imbalance (ERI) model, predicts that job strain will occur when workers do not feel adequately rewarded for the effort they invest in their work (Siegrist, 1996).

The two models have been used in several studies (most notably the Whitehall Studies and several large Scandinavian studies) that have explored the relationship between job strain and various health outcomes including CHD and mental health problems. The evidence they have yielded is equivocal; some found no relationship, while others found a doubling (or more) of the risk of negative health outcomes associated with those who reported higher levels of job strain (see Marmot et al, 2006 for a review of the evidence). Three of the leading figures in this field, Michael Marmot, Johannes Siegrist and Tores Theorell (2006) have drawn the conclusion that: 'Although "reporting bias" and "residual confounding" provide continuous challenges to this field of research, the overall evidence of links between work stress and health is nevertheless strong' (Marmot et al, 2006, p 121).

This conclusion has a high degree of face validity. It seems highly plausible that people in well-paid, secure jobs that are intrinsically satisfying, where the workload is sufficient to keep the individual active and engaged, but not so busy that they are constantly rushed off their feet, and where colleagues are friendly and supportive, will lead happier and healthier lives than those who are in poorly paid, insecure jobs that combine a heavy workload of dull and uninteresting work, where managers and colleagues are unsupportive or coercive.

The problem is that the 'good job' and the 'bad job' are ideal types. In real life, jobs have good and bad characteristics that can fluctuate over time. Moreover, the relative goodness or badness of a job is determined by far more than its objective characteristics. Leaving aside personality traits, genetic dispositions and negative experiences outside the workplace, the appraisal of the relative merits of a job may be shaped by the direction of change over time. For example, imagine two jobs. Job A has a heavier workload and poorer working conditions than job B, but over time the workload of job A eases slightly and working conditions improve a little, while in job B workload increases a little and working conditions deteriorate somewhat. Even after these changes, job B may still have objectively lower workload and better working conditions than job A, but will it be appraised as such by those working in job B? Not only that, but will those in job B not experience higher levels of distress, anxiety and depression than those in job A? Finally, if this distress and anxiety continues over time, might those in job A not experience higher levels of negative health outcomes than those in job B, even though their actual workload and working conditions remain objectively better? And might not all of these relationships be influenced by the way in which the employers manage the process of change, or by the extent to which those in job A compare their experiences with those of workers in job C who have experienced a substantially worse change of circumstances?

Stress theory (including the DCS and ERI models) lacks the conceptual and methodological apparatus to adequately explore these possibilities, but that has not stopped the proponents of work stress theory from trying to do so. It is towards these attempts to salvage the work stress model that we now turn.

Methodological attempts to salvage the paradigm

Despite its widespread acceptance, the discourse of work stress has not been immune to criticism (Briner and Reynolds, 1993; Doublet, 2000; Wainwright and Calnan, 2002; Patmore, 2006). Proponents of work stress theory have rarely engaged directly with these criticisms in print (see Siegrist, 2000 and Cooper and Dewe versus Wainwright, 2004 for two notable exceptions), although they have attempted to find methodological solutions to the problems raised. These methodological efforts have attempted to preserve the conceptual framework of work stress, rather than seriously addressing the conceptual problems with it. They have tended to focus on four areas: the subjective nature of appraisals (the tendency for people doing the same job to give very different appraisals of characteristics like demands and control); the role of negative affect as a confounding variable (the tendency for miserable people to give gloomy appraisals of work characteristics and mental health); the direction of causality (the possibility that psychiatrically distressed people might work less efficiently with the result that their workload backs up and they are granted less control over their work); and selection bias (the possibility that people with poor mental health in adolescence might be selected into jobs with poor work characteristics).

The Finnish Public Sector Study (Kouvonen et al, 2008) attempted to tackle the problem of the subjective nature of appraisals by aggregating appraisals of work characteristics across work groups, that is, small groups of workers were asked to individually appraise the level of social capital in their workplace, and these appraisals were then combined to produce an average for the group. This is a sensible strategy, as one would expect it to balance out the influence of individuals who gave an unduly pessimistic appraisal due to negative affect. When individual appraisals were correlated with antidepressant use it was found that those reporting low levels of workplace social capital were more likely to use antidepressants than those reporting low levels of social capital (odds ratio 1.36). However, when the analysis was repeated using aggregated appraisals of social support, this relationship completely disappeared; that is, workers in the low social capital group were no more likely to take antidepressants than those in the high social support group. This supports the criticism that the subjective nature of individual appraisals and negative affect can confound the relationship between work characteristics and poor mental health. However, even if the findings had been different and the relationship between social capital and antidepressant use had also been found in the analysis using aggregated data, it still would not be reasonable to conclude that the subjective nature of appraisals is not an important problem, because appraisals of this kind are fundamentally social – that is, they are influenced by interaction within the workplace social network. Put another way, how people appraise their work characteristics may be influenced by what their colleagues think of their job.

The social nature of appraisal also undermines attempts to use external assessors to calibrate job strain, rather than relying on workers' own appraisals. The Whitehall II study adopted this technique and found that the relationship between job strain and CHD remained even when job strain was independently assessed (Marmot et al, 2006). However, what is it that 'independent' assessors are actually assessing? The implication is that there are objective indicators of job demands, job control and social support that the assessor can access, when in reality their assessments are likely to be based on the extent to which groups of workers enact job strain, that is, the extent to which they present themselves as experiencing heavy workload, or low social support and so on. These enactments may well be based on workers' individual or collective appraisals, which again are subjective. In addition, independent assessors are themselves immersed in a broader set of cultural beliefs and normative expectations about the characteristics of different jobs. For example, the notion that life as a junior civil servant in the lower echelons of the state bureaucracy entails monotony, boredom and little opportunity to use personal discretion may be a deeply embedded cultural theme, in which case it would not be surprising if assessors steeped in that cultural narrative 'found' evidence of low job control when conducting their assessments.

A third strategy for tackling the subjective nature of appraisals has entailed doing away with them altogether and using objective indicators of job strain and health outcomes. One of the more sophisticated studies to adopt this strategy was the Work and Health in Finnish Hospital Personnel Study (Virtanen et al, 2008). Hospitals participating in the study routinely collected data on bed occupancy (sum of inpatient days divided by the number of beds available), and this variable was correlated with psychiatric illness absence and purchase of prescribed antidepressants. The researchers found a dose–response relationship between the degree of overcrowding (bed occupancy in increments above 85%) and depression-related sickness absence and the purchase of antidepressants. By conducting longitudinal multilevel analyses, the researchers were also able to address issues relating to selection bias and the direction of causality, by demonstrating a higher likelihood of starting a new antidepressant treatment after each six-month period of overcrowding.

Although the Work and Health in Finnish Hospital Personnel Study avoided the problem of subjective appraisals by adopting objective measures, it does not follow that the apparent relationship between the input variable (overcrowding) and the output variables (sickness absence for depression and purchase of antidepressants) is not mediated by social factors or the subjective nature of workers' appraisals. It may be that the problematisation of bed occupancy – its definition as 'overcrowding' – depends on the infringement of collectively negotiated workload norms – that is, what people define as an acceptable workload may itself be subjective and negotiated within the work group, rather than reflecting an objective point beyond which people cannot cope. Similarly, the response to this perception of heavy workload may also reflect group norms relating to illness behaviour; that is, there is nothing pre-ordained about the decision to take sickness absence or antidepressants in response to perceived increases in workload, and alternative strategies might include complaining to managers, involving the trade union, or simply rolling up one's sleeves and getting on with the work. There may be any number of cultural, structural or organisational factors that determine the course of action that will be taken. Work stress theorists are not able to address these issues because they are wedded to a stimulus–response model that sees human behaviour in terms of an unmediated response to objective conditions. They lack the conceptual insight to fully engage with the social dimension that mediates the relationship between working conditions and illness behaviour.

The struggle to defend the work stress model against its critics mirrors Thomas Kuhn's account of the revolutionary nature of scientific change:

> Mopping up operations are what engage most scientists throughout their careers. They constitute what I am here calling normal science....That enterprise seems an attempt to force nature into the pre-formed and relatively inflexible box that the paradigm supplies. No part of the aim of normal

science is to call forth new sorts of phenomena; indeed those that will not fit the box are often not seen at all. Nor do scientists aim to invent new theories, and they are often intolerant of those invented by others. (Kuhn, 1962, pp 23-4)

For Kuhn, the period of normal science continues until the prevailing paradigm and the theories it gives rise to collapse under the weight of contradictory evidence and conceptual weaknesses and a new paradigm emerges that has greater explanatory power than the one that preceded it. The rest of this chapter attempts to sketch out the broad contours of a new post-work stress paradigm, but first we present evidence that the old paradigm is beginning to lose its grip on the popular discourse of work and health.

Evidence of the fall

Despite extensive attempts to salvage the work stress model by methodological finesse, it remains conceptually flawed and unable to adequately grasp the complex relationship between experiences at work and their impact on mental and physical health. Even at the level of personal experience, many people are likely to find difficulty in accepting the claim that stress is simply another occupational hazard that affects the individual *in the same way* that, say, exposure to a dangerous chemical or a fall from a ladder might affect the body. Although the popular discourse of work stress remains the dominant narrative through which negative experiences at work are understood and made sense of, it is possible to detect a small but growing strand of incredulity towards its central claims and explanations.

There is even some evidence that work stress may be losing its grip on the popular imagination and on government agencies. Figure 9.2 shows that the annual number of major mentions of work stress in UK newspapers rose sharply in the late 1990s and the first two years of the new millennium, but has fallen from a high point in 2002.

Similarly, the government's Health and Safety Executive (HSE) had a keen interest in the work stress phenomenon throughout the 1990s, setting targets to reduce the incidence of work stress by 20% and the number of working days lost from work-related stress by 30%. Both targets were to be achieved by 2010 and the HSE implemented a 'management standards' programme comprising guidance for managers, dissemination of good practice and promotion of interventions in order to meet this target. However, as Figures 9.3 and 9.4 indicate, both variables remained fairly constant between 2001 and 2008.

Figure 9.2: Major mentions of work stress in UK newspapers, 1988-2008

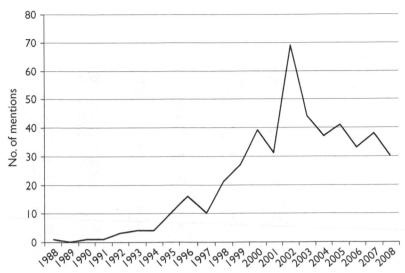

Source: LexisNexis

Figure 9.3: Estimated incidence of stress, depression or anxiety caused by work

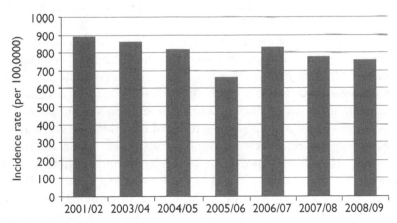

Source: Labour Force Survey

The HSE is the government agency with prime responsibility for protecting workers against hazards in the workplace, so it is significant that following the limited success of the management standards approach to tackling work stress, the HSE appears to be losing interest in what remains the major work-related health problem. In its 2001 strategy document, work stress is mentioned 55 times, but, in the 2009

Figure 9.4: Estimated average working days lost due to stress, anxiety or depression caused by work

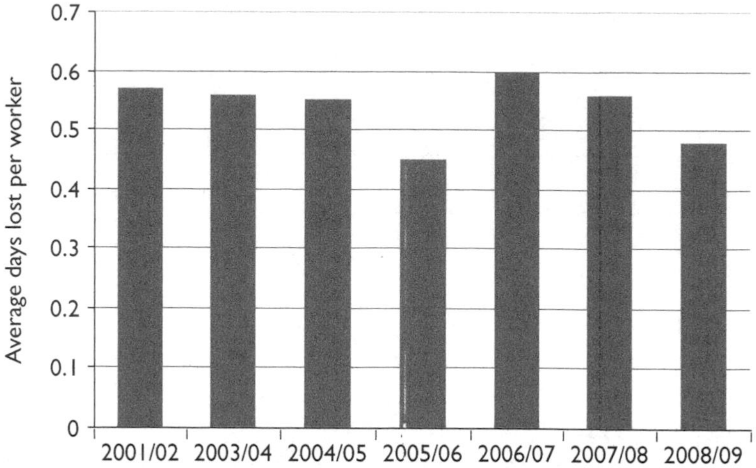

Source: Labour Force Survey

strategy, it receives not a single mention (HSC, 2001; HSE, 2009). Indeed, the illustration on the cover of the 2009 strategy document shows a stick-man with a broken leg, symbolising perhaps a return to occupational health's traditional domain of physical injury and a shift away from the vagaries of the psychosocial model.

It would be premature to conclude from the above evidence that work stress is diminishing in terms of its prevalence, but although many workers continue to 'feel stressed', the explanatory model of work stress appears to be losing traction, both as an academic paradigm and as a guide to effective policy and practice. Our argument is that this tendency, coupled with the conceptual and methodological problems we have described, indicates a fundamental crisis in the discourse of work stress that cannot be resolved by minor methodological innovations or conceptual tweaks to the prevailing approach. What is required is a fundamentally different way of thinking about the relationships between work, emotions, health and illness. We now argue that notion of 'wellbeing at work' offers the opportunity to build a new post work stress paradigm; but what does wellbeing mean?

Towards a new paradigm

The notion of wellbeing has a long history in public health circles, often as a vehicle for criticising the 'biomedical model', by which is meant the approach to ameliorating physical pathology that focuses on biology and medical intervention. Thus, in 1946, the World Health Organization (WHO) strove to redefine health as 'a state of complete physical, mental and social wellbeing and not merely the absence of disease or infirmity' (MacKenzie, 1946). It was not until the mid-1970s that the WHO's early conception of wellbeing began to have a significant impact on health policy and practice, with the WHO/ UNICEF Health for All by the Year 2000 initiative launched at Alma Ata in 1977 providing a defining moment in the rise of the New Public Health (Ashton and Seymour, 1988).

Since then, two strands have emerged within policies and practices that aim to enhance wellbeing. First came the implementation of health promotion strategies to encourage the adoption of 'healthy lifestyle' choices relating to diet, exercise, sexual behaviour and a range of other behaviours and activities thought to influence health outcomes (Fitzpatrick, 2001). More recently, a second strand has developed around the enhancement of 'subjective wellbeing', encapsulating a broad range of emotional and psychological states including low self-esteem, happiness and, inevitably, stress (Layard, 2005; Warr, 2007).

Importantly, for our purposes, these themes became interwoven in the current work, health and wellbeing agenda that has emerged from Dame Carol Black's review of the health needs of the working-age population and the government's response to that review (Black, 2008; DWP and DH, 2008). Where the discourse of work stress pathologises the workplace, seeing it as a source of mental and physical harm (Furedi, 1999), the Black review presents evidence of the benefits for mental and physical health that accrue from employment (Waddell and Burton, 2006; Black, 2008). This marks a fundamental philosophical shift, away from the notion of a fixed limit to human endurance that it is claimed work routinely pushes people beyond, towards a recognition that employment plays a central role in the fulfilment of human potential and aspiration.

The new wellbeing at work agenda provides a public intellectual space in which the problematic discourse of work stress may be set aside in favour of a new paradigm, but, as always, change of this kind brings with it strengths, weaknesses, opportunities and threats (SWOTs). We now present a brief SWOT analysis of the prevailing notion of wellbeing.

The WHO declaration serves to remind us that there is more to being well than simply not being physically ill, and that when people are ill this may reflect social and psychological factors as well as physical ones. However, by broadening the concept of health to include psychological and social wellbeing, the WHO declaration inadvertently transformed the pursuit of wellbeing into a health issue, rather than a political or economic concern. The intention may have been to demedicalise health policy, but the outcome was to bring new areas of everyday life within the purview of health policy.

The problem with this is that it may conflate health and wellbeing; that is, wellbeing may be viewed as a dimension of health, rather than an independent category that may have contradictory behavioural imperatives. For instance, rather than positing wellbeing as a synonym for health, we might define it in terms of the Aristotelian notion of 'the good life' or eudaimonia (Aristotle, 1962). Central to this distinction is the management of health risks and the tendency for individuals to engage in activities that might have adverse health consequences in order to achieve the emotional rewards that such activities confer – the off-piste skier, the soldier going off to war, the marathon runner straining to achieve a personal best, and the worker putting in long-hours of intense work in order to achieve a career goal, may all be risking their health in order to achieve a sense of subjective wellbeing.

If it is accepted that health and wellbeing are distinct categories and that there may on occasion be a trade-off between health risk and subjective wellbeing, there is a strong moral argument that this trade-off should be made by the individual rather than by an external agency. To give a concrete example, policies that aim to cap the length of the working week are often justified on the grounds that they will improve health and wellbeing (by reducing job strain). However, this overlooks the financial and emotional rewards that hard work and career advancement may bring, hence the necessity of including an opt-out clause in work time legislation to enable employees to waive this right.

The case for an individualised approach to the pursuit of wellbeing (or happiness – Murray, 1988) is further enhanced when the subjective nature of appraisal is considered. The appraisal of work characteristics, such as the magnitude of job demands, is highly subjective, as is the self-appraisal of resilience and the capacity to cope with job demands. From this perspective, personal volition and choice should be central to the promotion of wellbeing at work; let individuals decide for themselves how demanding their job is and whether they are willing and able to commit the time and effort required to meet those demands. It is this internal conversation (Archer, 2003), in which individuals reflect on how hard they are willing to push themselves and what they are prepared to sacrifice in order to achieve their goals, that defines our notion of resilience and agency.

Reconstructing notions of wellbeing at work around individual agency is an important corrective to the overly deterministic discourse of work stress that sees the individual as a passive victim of objective workplace conditions whose thoughts and preferences are irrelevant in determining their behaviour or their wellbeing. However, there are two problems with this approach. First, it assumes that the commitment of time and effort by the worker is freely chosen, for example, that he chooses to work long hours in order to enjoy the satisfaction of achieving career goals, when in fact there may be structural and organisational factors that demand increased work effort and longer hours, without the reward of achieving career goals. Second, as we have argued above, the appraisal of work characteristics and decisions about how to respond to them, for example, whether to engage in illness behaviour, may also be conditioned by social factors, including work place norms, interaction and negotiation with work colleagues and the broader social network, and by broader cultural narratives like the discourse of work stress.

In short, wellbeing at work is neither an unmediated response to objective working conditions (as the discourse of work stress implies), but neither is it an entirely individual phenomenon that can be fully explained in terms of individual preferences and positive thinking. Work does have an objective reality, but this reality is mediated by the lived experience of the worker as he appraises his experiences through interaction within his social network and a broader cultural milieu. In Figure 9.5 we have attempted to model a post–work–stress paradigm of wellbeing at work.

At the centre of the model is the individual self, embodied with genetic predispositions and relatively fixed personality traits, but also a conscious subject making sense of his lived experiences and making

Figure 9.5: Social determinants of wellbeing and illness behaviour

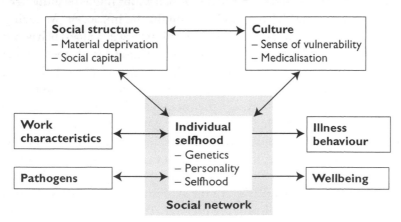

choices about how to act. Work characteristics affect the individual, but so do other factors, including pathogens, the social structure and broad cultural narratives that influence behaviour. Crucially, these factors do not affect the individual directly, but are mediated by the social network both at work and in the broader community. This process of mediation entails the individual making sense of his experiences of the external world through interaction with significant others and selecting from the (sometimes narrow) range of responses that these external factors determine. For our purposes, there are two important outputs from this model. The first is illness behaviour; for example, in response to, say a rapid increase in workload, a worker may respond by taking sick leave or seeking medical help (see Wainwright, 2008 for a review of the sociological literature on illness behaviour). The second is wellbeing, in which the individual exhibits resilience, overcomes negative experiences and achieves a high degree of emotional satisfaction and contentment.

There are a number of important things to note about the relationships posited in the model. First is the high degree of contingency or indeterminacy in the relationships between the input and output variables. This is not a simple stimulus-response or cause-and-effect model, in which the same input variables must inevitably lead to the same outcomes. For example, the same array of objective working conditions may lead to a high degree of wellbeing and a low degree of illness behaviour, or to the reverse, depending on the other factors in the model and, crucially, how the individual invests them with meaning within the context of his social network. Second, the model does not ignore the potency of external factors in conditioning the array of outputs. For example, severe physical trauma may be a very strong predictor of illness behaviour and might also predict a negative outcome in terms of wellbeing. However, even with severe physical trauma, the degree and extent of illness behaviour might be influenced by the other factors in the model, as might the impact on wellbeing. Finally, it is worth noting that the relationship between illness behaviour and wellbeing may function as a zero-sum relationship; that is, a higher degree of wellbeing might generate a low degree of illness behaviour and vice versa, but this relationship is not absolute and depends on the configuration of other factors in the model. Thus it is not impossible to imagine scenarios in which an individual exhibits high self-esteem and high levels of illness behaviour, or indeed low levels of both outputs.

A key question in assessing this new paradigm is whether it overcomes the conceptual and methodological problems of the work stress approach. Our initial criticism of the discourse of work stress was that it was largely ahistorical, or more precisely that its claim that the work stress epidemic was purely a response to a broad worsening of working conditions following the economic slump of the mid-1970s, did not fit with a broader historical analysis that shows far worse working conditions prior to that date, but no evidence of an earlier epidemic of work stress. The new paradigm includes not only structural change, but also cultural changes, including medicalisation and a heightened sense of vulnerability (Furedi, 2004) and the way that these factors are interpreted and made sense of within social networks. There is a rich vein of sociological literature on the cultural influences on orientation to work, including classic accounts such as Weber's *The Protestant ethic and the spirit of capitalism* (1965) and Goldthorpe and colleagues' *The affluent worker* (1968) (see Watson, 2008 for a useful review of this literature). The inclusion of these factors allows the shift from a realist ontology to a social constructionist approach – thus the work stress epidemic can be recognised not just as an unmediated response to objective work characteristics, but also as a discursive formation, that is, as a cultural narrative through which people make sense of the world and choose how to act.

A second criticism was that work stress is poorly specified and refers to a wide range of stressors, emotional states and mental and physical health problems. This is a problem if our interest lies in building an epidemiological model, where specificity and clear causative relationships are essential. The new model recognises that the relationship between working life and health and wellbeing cannot be adequately grasped by the methods of epidemiology, which are derived from the biological reductionism of the natural sciences, because these relationships are mediated by consciousness and subjectivity. Thus the new paradigm entails a shift away from positivism towards an interpretivist epistemology. In this sense, the new paradigm does not solve the old problem of trying to give a more specific definition of work stress variables and a clearer account of the relationships between them; rather, it recognises that this endeavour was always a fool's errand.

A third problem with the work stress approach is that it fails to adequately acknowledge the role of subjectivity in the appraisal of work characteristics, leading to a series of unsuccessful attempts to move away from self-report data towards more objective measures of job strain. Again, rather than treating subjectivity as a confounding variable that must be controlled or excluded, the new paradigm recognises that subjectivity is absolutely central to understanding the relationship between work and wellbeing, making subjective appraisals an important object of study in their own right.

Finally, we criticised the work stress model for its assumption of mono-causality, that is, that there is a unilinear relationship between work characteristics and emotional wellbeing and its health correlates. This assumption has led epidemiologists into various attempts to establish the direction of causality and exclude the possibility of selection bias. The new paradigm punctures the myth of mono-causality, recognising that the relationship between work characteristics, illness behaviour and wellbeing is always contingent on a wide range of other factors – individual, organisational, social and cultural – that cannot simply be factored out to reveal a unilinear relationship. Methodologically, the new paradigm calls for recognition of complexity, rather than reductionism.

In conclusion, the new paradigm of work and wellbeing that we have posited entails a fundamental ontological and epistemological shift. The relationship between work and wellbeing is fundamentally different to, say, the relationship between tobacco smoking and lung cancer, and requires a different methodology in order to understand it. In the past, we have asked the wrong questions about the relationship between work and wellbeing and sought methodological innovations to answer questions that are fundamentally unanswerable. The new paradigm raises a new set of questions about the social aspects of appraisals, their impact on resilience and illness behaviour, and what can be done to promote wellbeing at work given the implications of the new approach. These questions are barely formulated, much less operationalised, and this new research agenda will doubtless raise methodological and conceptual problems of its own. However, it does offer a route out of the various culs de sac of the work stress discourse. A first step on this pathway is to agree a moratorium on use of the term work stress.

Further reading

Briner, R.B. and Reynolds, S. (1993) 'Bad theory and bad practice in occupational stress', *The Occupational Psychologist*, vol 19, pp 8-13.

Green, F. (2006) *Demanding work: The paradox of job quality in the affluent economy*, Princeton, NJ: Princeton University Press.

Karasek, R. and Theorell, T. (1990) *Healthy work: Stress, productivity and the reconstruction of working life*, New York, NY: Basic Books.

Wainwright, D. (2008) 'Illness behaviour and the discourse of health', in D. Wainwright (ed) *A sociology of health*, London: Sage Publications.

Wainwright, D. and Calnan, M. (2002) *Work stress: The making of a modern epidemic*, Buckingham: Open University Press.

References

Archer, M.S. (2003) *Structure, agency and the internal conversation*, Cambridge: Cambridge University Press.

Aristotle (1962) *The Nicomachean ethics* (translated by Martin Oswald), New York, NY: Bobs–Merrill Company.

Ashton, J. and Seymour, H. (1988) *The New Public Health*, Milton Keynes: Open University Press.

Black, C. (2008) *Working for a healthier tomorrow*, London: The Stationery Office.

Briner, R.B. and Reynolds, S. (1993) 'Bad theory and bad practice in occupational stress', *The Occupational Psychologist*, vol 19, pp 8-13.

Burke, R.J. and Cooper, C.L. (2000) *The organisation in crisis: Downsizing, restructuring and privatisation*, Oxford: Blackwell.

Cooper, C. and Dewe, P. versus Wainwright, D. (March 2004) 'Managing workplace stress', *Science & Public Affairs*, pp 4-5, www.britishscienceassociation.org/NR/rdonlyres/F1FD95BE-DBF6-4A8D-8E51-020B8C53F08C/0/4106_SPA_March_04.pdf

Davey Smith, G., Dorling, D. and Shaw, M. (2001) *Poverty, inequality and health in Britain 1800-2000: A reader*, Bristol: The Policy Press.

Doublet, S. (2000) *The stress myth*, Chesterfield, MO: Science & Humanities Press.

DWP and DH (Department for Work and Pensions and Department of Health) (2008) *Improving health and work: Changing lives*, London: The Stationery Office.

Fitzpatrick, M. (2001) *The tyranny of health: Doctors and the regulation of lifestyle*, London: Routledge.

Furedi, F. (1999) 'Diseasing the workplace', *Occupational Health Review*, November, pp 26-9.

Goldthorpe, J.H., Lockwood, D., Bechhofer, F. and Platt, J. (1968) *The affluent worker: Industrial attitudes and behaviour*, Cambridge: Cambridge University Press.

Green, F. (2001) '"It's been a hard day's night": the concentration and intensification of work in late 20th century Britain', *British Journal of Industrial Relations*, vol 39, no 1, pp 53-80.

Green, F. (2006) *Demanding work: The paradox of job quality in the affluent economy*, Princeton, NJ: Princeton University Press.

Hobsbawm, E.J. (1968) *Industry and empire*, Harmondsworth: Penguin.

HSC (Health and Safety Commission) (2001) *Strategic plan 2001/2004*, London: HSE Books.

HSE (Health and Safety Executive) (2009) *The health and safety of Great Britain: Be part of the solution*, London: HSE.

Karasek, R. and Theorell, T. (1990) *Healthy work: Stress, productivity and the reconstruction of working life*, New York, NY: Basic Books.

Kouvonen, A., Oksanen, T., Vahtera, J., Stafford, M., Wilkinson, R., Schneider, J., Vaananen, A., Virtanen, M., Cox, S.J., Pentti, J., Elovainio, M. and Kivimaki, M. (2008) 'Low workplace social capital as a predictor of depression: the Finnish Public Sector Study', *American Journal of Epidemiology*, vol 167, no 10, pp 1143-51.

Kuhn, T.S. (1962) *The structure of scientific revolutions*, Chicago, IL: University of Chicago Press.

Layard, R. (2005) *Happiness: Lessons from a new science*, London: Allen Lane.

Lazarus, R. and Folkman, S. (1984) *Stress, appraisal and coping*, New York, NY: Springer.

MacKenzie, M.D. (1946) 'The World Health Organisation', *British Medical Journal*, 21 September, pp 428-30.

Marmot, M., Siegrist, J. and Theorell, T. (2006) 'Health and the psychosocial environment at work', in M. Marmot and R. Wilkinson (eds) *Social determinants of health* (3rd edn), Oxford: Oxford University Press.

Meyerson, D.E. (1998) 'Feeling stressed and burned out: a feminist reading and re-visioning of stress-based emotions within medicine and organization science', *Organization Science*, vol 9, no 1, pp 103-18.

Murray, C. (1988) *In pursuit of happiness and good government*, London: Simon & Schuster.

ONS (Office for National Statistics) (2009) 'The Labour Force Survey', www.statistics.gov.uk/statbase/Source.asp?vlnk=358&More=Y#general

Paris, J. (2010) 'Biopsychosocial models and psychiatric diagnosis', in T. Millon, R.F. Kreuger and E. Simonsen (eds) *Contemporary directions in psychopathology: Scientific foundations of the DSM-V and ICD-11*, New York, NY: Guilford Press.

Patmore, A. (2006) *The truth about stress*, London: Atlantic Books.

Siegrist, J. (1996) 'Adverse health effects of high-effort/low-reward conditions', *Journal of Occupational Health Psychology*, vol 1, pp 27-41.

Siegrist, J. (2000) 'Work stress and beyond', *European Journal of Public Health*, vol 10, no 3, pp 233-4.

Stansfeld, S.A. and Marmot, M.G. (eds) (2002) *Stress and the heart: Psychosocial pathways and coronary heart disease*, London: BMJ Books.

Virtanen, M., Pentti, J., Vahtera, J., Ferrie, J.E., Stansfeld, S.A., Helenius, H., Elovainio, M., Honkonen, T., Terho, K., Oksanen, T. and Kivimäki, M. (2008) 'Overcrowding in hospital wards as a predictor of antidepressant treatment among hospital staff', *American Journal of Psychiatry*, vol 165, pp 1482-6.

Waddell, G. and Burton, A.K. (2006) *Is work good for your health and wellbeing?*, London: The Stationery Office.

Wainwright, D. (2008) 'Illness behaviour and the discourse of health', in D. Wainwright (ed) *A sociology of health*, London: Sage Publications.

Wainwright, D. and Calnan, M. (2002) *Work stress: The making of a modern epidemic*, Buckingham: Open University Press.

Warr, P. (2007) *Work, happiness and unhappiness*, London: Lawrence Erlbaum Associates.

Watson, T.J. (2008) *Sociology, work and industry* (5th edn), London: Routledge.

Weber, M. (1965) *The Protestant ethic and the spirit of capitalism*, London: Allen and Unwin.

TEN

'Work Ability': a practical model for improving the quality of work, health and wellbeing across the life-course?

Tony Maltby

This chapter offers a descriptive, yet critical, overview of a holistic approach to managing health and wellbeing of employees that has been developed in Finland from the 1980s by the Finnish Institute of Occupational Health (FIOH). Known as the Work Ability model (Ilmarinen, 2010), it attempts to integrate all aspects of the health and wellbeing of individuals and should be seen as a preventative approach to the management of a broad range of health issues in the workplace. Thus it could extend the quality working life of all adults, but more especially (and its initial purpose) those over 50, generally described in the literature as 'older workers'. It is offered here as an example of an integrated yet scientifically based approach to the improvement of health and wellbeing over the life-course that could be introduced into the United Kingdom (UK). It would build on the work of the Health, Work and Wellbeing strategy led by Dame Carol Black during the last Labour administration (see Black, 2008) (to be discussed later).

This chapter first provides a description of the Finnish approach and a brief background to its development as a method within what has been termed 'age management'. It then considers how it might be applied in the UK context, given the policy shift of raising the state pension age, and thus (potentially) extending the time spent in employment. Fundamental to the method is the promotion of 'active ageing' (see Walker, 2002; WHO, 2002) and the productive and quality-led extension of working life. This assumes that all individuals want to, and indeed need to, extend their working lives and certainly this may not always be the case. However, for a substantial number, continuing to work may be a financial necessity, as well as a desirable goal in some cases (Smeaton et al, 2008). Additionally, it has been demonstrated through scientifically rigorous studies that the Work

Ability approach can lead to a better quality of retirement over the longer term (Tuomi et al, 2001; Gould et al, 2008). Other research evidence has demonstrated that employees value work for a range of reasons, including intrinsic interest and sense of purpose, the ability to use skills and knowledge acquired over a lifetime, social status and self-respect, and social engagement with colleagues and workmates, customers and partners (McNair and Flynn, 2006; Waddell and Burton, 2006). Nevertheless, as contributors to this volume have demonstrated, work can also lead to negative impacts (see, for example, Griffiths, 2007; Hill et al, 2007), especially if it is poorly managed and organised at the level of the enterprise – where people are most affected. Such 'bad' work is also one of the major factors in shortening the working lives of individuals, affecting their future quality of life, their health and wellbeing. This is often a direct outcome of poor quality work and workplace design (see, for example, Phillipson and Smith, 2005; McNair and Flynn, 2006) and poor management practices. Some of the worse effects of such 'bad' work have been ameliorated over the past century in most modern economies through the implementation, enforced by statute, of a variety of what have been called 'health and safety' and 'equal opportunities' provisions. Implementation of a Work Ability approach could, it is suggested, be implemented in a similar fashion and for similar reasons – to improve the health and working conditions of the working population.

It is, therefore, important to both individuals and enterprises how extensions to a good-quality working life might be pursued (Smeaton and Vegeris, 2009). For example, a high proportion of older people say they would only consider a longer working life on a part-time or 'flexible' basis (Vickerstaff et al, 2008; Smeaton and Vegeris, 2009). Over the period 1992 to 2009, the percentage of those in employment over state pension age has risen from 8% to 12%, but with this increase comprising mainly those working on a part-time basis (Dini, 2009; ONS, 2009). Yet, whatever method people select, the actual employment experience is central to any consideration of improving the quality of work and, as a result, the health and wellbeing of the individual. As argued elsewhere (Maltby, 2011), giving greater attention to the quality of work, *and* to health and wellbeing, must be a major priority for economic and social policy. Policy measures aimed at changing 'early exit' to 'late exit' – that is, extending working lives – should be sensitive to the actual processes and organisation of work, to flows out of the labour market and to the quality of the work undertaken in order to help retain staff – 'older workers' in particular.

The Finnish approach

The traditional approach to occupational health in the UK has been based on a largely individualistic paradigm of health and illness. This approach has tended to emphasise the failings of the individual, adopting primarily a biomedical, rather than a social or biopsychosocial model of health (see Engel, 1977; Navarro, 1978; Townsend and Davidson, 1981; Borrell-Carrió et al, 2004). Crudely, a biomedical approach views the body as a machine comprising replaceable parts that can be repaired (that is, by drugs) or replaced (that is, through surgery) when they 'fail'. In contrast, a biopsychosocial model recognises that many of the (occupational health and work–related) difficulties and causes of ill health relate not to the individual worker but to the work environment including the organisation's structures and practices and their impact on the individual, set within a personal and socioeconomic milieu.

Biopsychosocial perspectives, in contrast with the biomedical approach, emphasise the importance of social factors influencing health and illness, drawing in particular on the World Health Organization model of 'active ageing' as a guiding principle. This approach has been defined as:

> ... the process of optimizing opportunities for health, participation and security in order to enhance quality of life as people age... It allows people to realize their potential for physical, social, and mental well being throughout the life course and to participate in society according to their needs, desires and capacities, while providing them with adequate protection, security and care when they require assistance.... (WHO, 2002, p 12)

It requires that the prevailing approach is both preventative and empowering (Walker, 2002), reducing the need for reactive interventions when problems have already occurred – a common feature of the biomedical model (see Rose, 2008). Poor performance, poor health and premature retirement may be consequences of, for example, poor work design and management practices, rather than some inevitable failing of the worker (such as illness and/or a disability). Confirmation of this has come from quantitative as well as qualitative research into older people's attitudes to work and retirement (Humphrey, et al, 2003; Irving et al, 2005; Maltby, 2007).

It is clear from the evidence presented in this volume and elsewhere that adoption of a biopsychosocial model would have considerable advantages for individuals, enterprises and the economy. Much of this external evidence derives from work carried out by Finnish investigators (see Ilmarinen, 2005; Gould et al, 2008). Indeed, work carried out in Finland over more than three decades (Ilmarinen, 2010) demonstrates that such an approach is possible and practicable, and merits serious exploration in a UK context. It has been piloted and used in several countries within and beyond the EU, including the Netherlands,[1] Germany, Sweden, Norway, Austria, Brazil and Portugal. There has been a large-scale research study (see http://respect.iccs.ntua. gr/index.html) that employed this conceptual framework. A European-wide review led by the Institute of Employment Research at Warwick University (Lindley et al, 2006) documents this work and reports on several case studies where the approach has been implemented as well as producing a number of recommendations. These demonstrate and conclude that Work Ability is not only robust but also culture-free, thus allowing international collaboration and comparison. Additionally, and more significantly for the UK, it is currently being evaluated for use in Australia (Taylor et al, 2010), bearing in mind the cultural and other historical ties between the two countries. Yet Work Ability, as an approach, has not, to date, been systematically evaluated or piloted in the UK, although there have been several small-scale investigations. This is despite the Finnish EU presidencies of 1999 and 2006 promoting the concepts of Work Ability and age management throughout the EU.

The Work Ability 'house'

Economic and demographic concerns surfacing in Finland during the 1980s were major factors behind the development of the Work Ability approach (see Ilmarinen, 1999). During this period, the Finnish government identified the rapidity of population ageing in comparison with other EU countries and the problems this might bring for the economy. Labour force projections indicated that the proportion of workers aged 50 and over would move from being lower than the average for the EU15 in 1995 to being the highest (33%) by 2005, with this position continuing up until 2015 (Ilmarinen, 1999). The policy response was to seek methods to extend the working life of these older workers, while recognising that any extension was 'highly dependent upon [their] health, functional capacity, skills and working conditions ...' (Ilmarinen, 1999, p 16).

Consequentially, the FIOH (under Ilmarinen) undertook a research and development programme, focusing on older workers, to develop and test tools to support retaining people in the workforce for longer.

More recently, this has been extended to encompass the entire workforce in an effort to improve the quality of work experienced by all employees. The key tool is the Work Ability Index (WAI) (see next section and Tuomi et al, 1998), which is a measure described by Ilmarinen and his colleagues as a test of 'How good is the worker at present, in the near future, and how able is he or she to do his or her work with respect to the work demands, health and mental resources?' (Ilmarinen and Tuomi, 2004, p 2)

Based on the results from various research studies conducted by Ilmarinen and his colleagues over the past 30 years, work ability is described as having four dimensions:

- work organisation and leadership (environment, content and demands, community and organisation, management and leadership);
- values (attitudes and motivation);
- competence (knowledge and skills); and
- health (functional capacities).

These have been graphically represented as the work ability 'house' (see Figure 10.1). This framework attempts to reflect the importance and integration of each of these four dimensions, and, importantly, the role of external non-work-based factors influencing working performance and productivity, for example the family, relatives and friends, and society. An individual's resources form the central core of work ability, and comprise the first three floors:

- The first floor expresses the physical and mental health and functional capacity of an individual; the stronger this foundation floor the better the individual's work ability (Ilmarinen, 2005).
- The second tier involves the professional expertise and competences, knowledge and skill and their continual updating through, for example, lifelong learning.
- The third floor comprises the contributions made by personal values and attitudes, as well as those factors that motivate them, with positive attitudes enhancing work ability.
- The fourth floor consists of the work environment, the content and demands of that work, the work community (for example, the work-based 'team', office or factory community) and the work organisation. Supervision and management of individuals are also part of the fourth floor, which can be seen to be the heaviest, most dominant floor.

Figure 10.1: New model: work ability and environment

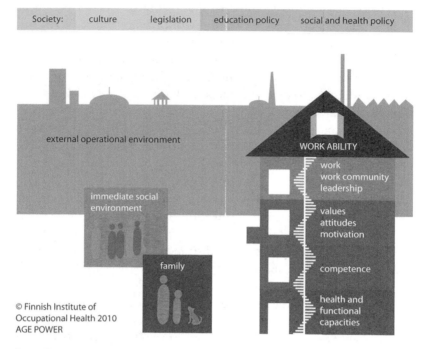

Society: culture   legislation   education policy   social and health policy

external operational environment

WORK ABILITY

work
work community
leadership

immediate social
environment

values
attitudes
motivation

family

competence

health and
functional
capacities

© Finnish Institute of
Occupational Health 2010
AGE POWER

Source: Finnish Institute of Occupational Health

Ilmarinen (2005, p 133) concludes that 'Work ability is primarily a question of balance between work and personal resources' – a balance between the fourth and the other three floors. Thus, work ability will deteriorate if the three lower floors are not in proportion with the size and functionality of this top floor. The importance of the role of good management practices in supporting workers has been demonstrated in longitudinal studies implementing the Work Ability model (Tuomi, 1997; Tuomi et al, 2001).

Importantly, the 'house' model emphasises that work ability is not separated from life outside work. In the immediate surroundings of the 'house' are the organisations that support a working life (for example occupational health care and health and safety) as well as the family and the close community (such as relatives, friends, acquaintances). The outermost layer represents societal structures, whose infrastructure (for example, social, educational, health and occupational policies and services) form the macro environment of WA (Ilmarinen and Tuomi, 2004, p 20; Ilmarinen, 2005, pp 132 onwards).

In the reports from longitudinal studies (see for example Ilmarinen and Tuomi, 2004; Ilmarinen, 2005; Gould et al, 2008), it is argued that if left unchecked, the core components of an individual's work ability often naturally decline during the life-course and a person's working career. This is a result not only of the commonly cited changes affecting many older workers, but also of the introduction of new technologies, the changing pace of work and the impact of a global economic pressures (ILO, 2006). Fundamentally, therefore, in order to maintain good work ability, it is imperative to 'strive for a safe balance between work and human resources' (Gould et al, 2008, p 20).

The Work Ability Index

In order to assess an individual's work ability – the long-term capacity to work in his or her present job – the Work Ability Index (WAI) was developed through a number of empirically based studies (Ilmarinen and Tuomi, 2004). The results can be used to design individual and workplace interventions that reduce premature withdrawal from the labour market and the natural decline mentioned earlier. Ilmarinen (2005, chapters 4, 5 and 6) describes some examples of these interventions, which are often offered as an integrated package and include, for example, better ergonomic design, better working practices, participation in adult education programmes, fitness programmes and so on. Overall, these attempt to ensure that the elements that make up the Work Ability 'house' are balanced and involve a 'methodological and purposeful range of actions taken in cooperation with the employer and employees' (Peltomäki et al, 2002; Ilmarinen, 2005, p 137).

Use of the WAI is therefore an integral part of what has been termed 'age management'. In simple terms, this is about managing people of different ages better, and is the means through which work ability, as measured by the WAI, is enhanced and then maintained. A more definitive description of age management that emphasises occupational health and work is as follows:

> Age management requires taking the employee's age and age related factors into account in their daily work management, work planning and work organisation; thus everyone – regardless of age – can achieve personal and organizational targets healthily and safely. (Ilmarinen, 2005, p 120)

And later in the same work Ilmarinen suggests:

> With good age management, work is planned and organized according to the resources of the personnel. Age

management also supports the development of employees' resources. It is not, however, rational or even possible to make all age groups similar. Age management emphasizes and utilizes strength in diversity and makes it a success factor for both the individual and the enterprise. The most noble and precious objective of age management is to ensure that employees have the prerequisites for a good life and that the enterprise has a good future. (Ilmarinen, 2005, p 234)

The evidence from the Finnish Work Ability programme, part of the country's National Programme on Ageing Workers 1998-2002, suggests that the systematic measurement of work ability, linked to improvements in age management, can lead to reductions in premature labour market withdrawal, as well as greater job satisfaction, improved health and raised productivity.

An individual WAI score is determined through a series of self-completed questions that examine seven key areas and offer an evaluative score through consideration of the physical and mental demands of work and the health and resources of the employee. The key seven areas are:

- Current work ability compared with the lifetime best and comprises the work ability score that is often used as a separate indicator of work ability (0-10 points).
- Work ability in relation to the demands of the job (2-10 points).
- Number of current diseases diagnosed by a physician (1-7 points).
- Estimated work impairment due to diseases (1-6 points).
- Sick leave during the past year (1-5 points).
- Own prognosis of work ability two years from now (1, 4 or 7 points).
- Mental resources (1-4 points) (Tuomi et al, 1998).

Through summation of the scores of the seven items listed, the overall WAI score can be calculated, resulting in a range of 7-59 points. This represents four levels of work ability from poor (7-27) through to moderate (28-36), good (37-43) and excellent (44-49) (Tuomi et al, 1998). The reliability of the WAI scores as measured by Chonbach's alpha has ranges from 0.78 to 0.83, indicating good reliability (Illmarinen and Tuomi, 2004; Gould et al, 2008). In research studies, good work ability was found to be positively associated with a high quality of work and enjoying one's job (Tuomi et al, 2001).

The development of the questionnaire and its validity was based on a longitudinal study of older municipal employees commencing in 1981 and repeated in 1985, 1991 and 1997 and involved clinical examination, observation at the workplace and correlation analysis (Tuomi et al, 1985; Ilmarinen, 1991; Ilmarinen et al, 1991; Tuomi et al, 1991; Tuomi, 1997). It was through such research that the predictive power of the WAI came to be realised, and thus demanded the application of a range of interventions that could improve or at least maintain the work ability of individuals. Not only was it demonstrated that an individual's work ability gradually and naturally declines with increasing age but also that younger and well-educated people perceived their work ability to be better than those who were older or had less education. Those who were married had higher work ability than those who were single or divorced. Interestingly, those in full-time employment perceived their work ability to be higher than those who were working part-time, and white-collar workers had higher scores than blue-collar workers. Agricultural workers gave the lowest estimate of their work ability (see Gould et al, 2008).

The WAI has been validated on a range of different research populations and within different types of enterprises, including some large ones, over a period of more than 30 years. It has been shown to accurately measure job satisfaction and depression, predict future levels of mental wellbeing and emotional exhaustion, predict active and meaningful life after retirement and identify the types of work that cause problems for older workers (Ilmarinen and Tuomi, 2004; Ilmarinen, 2005, p 78 onwards) before the need for a medical intervention. It is cheap and simple to administer, and produces reliable objective results. It examines both physical and psychological health and the relationship of the individual to the enterprise or workplace. When used on people in their mid-40s, it has been reported to predict the likelihood that an individual will withdraw prematurely from the labour market (Tuomi et al, 2001).

Since its publication in 1992, the WAI has been translated into 26 languages (Ilmarinen, 2010). Four international symposia have been held to develop and discuss the ideas, the most recent held in 2010 in Tampere, Finland. In 1989, promotion of the Work Ability model was incorporated into a national agreement between employers and trades unions in Finland and 80% of Finnish companies have made some use of the concepts. The FIOH is now engaged in a 28-year follow-up survey of the original municipal employees originally surveyed, a 10-year follow-up of the national surveys with the WAI (with aim of further developing the survey instruments) and development of various training and coaching tools (Ilmarinen, 2010).

The UK approach: the Health, Work and Wellbeing strategy

Launched in October, 2005, the Health, Work and Wellbeing strategy (HWWB) was a cross-government partnership between the Department for Work and Pensions, the Department of Health, the Health and Safety Executive and the health departments within the Scottish Executive and Welsh Assembly governments. The strategy was borne out of recognition that an overall 80% employment rate, which some thought as unachievable, would never be realised if all that was done was to support those who were already recipients of state benefits (OASPG, 2008). The policy argument had thus altered to suggest that there was '... a need to prevent people from falling out of work and needing to claim benefits in the first place' (OASPG, 2008). The basis of this policy shift was founded on the following set of statistics:

• 175 million working days a year lost to sickness absence, at a cost of £13 billion (Confederation of British Industry);
• 36 million working days a year (currently) lost to work-related sickness or injury (Health and Safety Executive);
• 2.7 million people (currently) claim incapacity benefits and 600,000 new people flow on each year;
• almost 1.5 million 50- to 59-year-olds say that they cannot work due to a health problem or disability (OASPG, 2008).

Such facts were widely known and discussed. Significantly, the key focus was on health and illness, for which read sickness and the management of the recorded levels along a downward trajectory. The strategy did not focus on a holistic conceptualisation of health and wellbeing, as in Finland, nor on the well-documented negative effects of employment that might affect health and wellbeing (see, for example, Humphrey et al, 2003; Irving et al, 2005; Waddell and Burton, 2006; Lindley et al, 2006). Importantly, and again in contrast with the Finnish approach, the implementation of the UK approach has often been neither preventative, holistic in approach, but *ex post* facto, dominated by biomedically based solutions, founded on an individualistic paradigm of health and illness. The evidence for this assessment is to be found within the Black (2008) report itself and the associated documentation. It states that the focus of the HWWB strategy is:

• to ensure that the general health of the working-age population improves;

- to prevent work–related illness and injury, but also to go further and use the workplace as an opportunity for general health improvement;
- to respond early when health problems arise – and, combined with this, ensure that the necessary interventions are easily and speedily available;
- to help people to better manage their conditions so that they can lead as full a life as possible;
- to ensure that appropriate rehabilitation support and workplace adaptations are available for those who have been out of work because of ill health, enabling them to make that leap back into work as soon as possible' (HSE, 2010).

It was argued that central to the achievement of these objectives, it would be necessary to engage with healthcare professionals, especially general practitioners (GPs), improve access to healthcare to resolve 'common health problems' and ensure the support of employers (OASPG, 2008). However, a key aspect of the strategy was a review, led by Dame Carol Black, of the health of the working-age population. This documented a variety of statistics, largely drawn from existing published government data, advancing the case for a heightened policy input into workplace health and wellbeing. It also recommended an integrated approach to the health of people of working age, asserting a more prominent role for occupational health and vocational rehabilitation professions. The report suggested that the new vision was based on:

- the prevention of illness and promotion of health and wellbeing;
- early intervention for those who develop a health condition; and
- an improvement in the health of those out of work – so that everyone with the potential to work has the support they need to do so (Black, 2008, p 9).

The first of these priorities is in keeping with the Finnish approach. Yet the report failed to document any methods as to how this strategy might be measured and implemented other than through the limited 'Fit for Work' scheme (see Black, 2008, pp 77-82 for details and to follow). Consultants to the HWWB, PricewaterhouseCoopers, did, however, design and implement a 'workplace wellbeing tool'. This allows individual enterprises to offer an econometric analysis of the costs and benefits of staff ill health, consider the economic returns of investment in a health and wellbeing programme that could be developed by example from existing initiatives, and the sharing and learning of best practice through UK-based case studies (HWWB, 2010). This suggests that the approach was left to each individual employer with little support from government. Yet the PricewaterHouse Coopers study, which also contained a literature review, ignored, in common with the Black report (2008), the extensive work of the FIOH and the well-tried and rigorously tested WAI approach. For a major review such as this, it would have been expected for some mention to be made of Work Ability, a programme that had been widely disseminated and publicised and had similar aims and objectives to those in the UK.

That the Black report did suggest the importance of prevention and the role of the workplace in supporting health and wellbeing, and indicated that health and wellbeing was not simply a medical issue (see Black, 2008, chapter 3) and that 'good health is good business' (Black, 2008, p 10), is to be welcomed. Yet the recommendations and their subsequent implementation suggest the opposite. The policy outcome for this vital element would be developed, it argued, through the high-profile fit-for-work (more accurately, Statement of Fitness to Work or 'fit note') certification process that replaced the 'sick note' (Medical Statement), delivered through the GP network from April 2010. This places the obligation on GPs to assess the work someone could do rather than what they could not do, and supports a biomedical approach to health and wellbeing, operating remotely from the workplace. The most recent iteration of this ideological approach to welfare is to be found within the 2011 Welfare Reform Bill currently (at time of writing) being discussed in Parliament. This maintains the similar, if less nuanced approach, of the previous Labour administration (see DSS, 1998, chapter 3). Labour developed the New Deal programmes as one of the mechanisms that provided incentives for people to move into paid employment (Maltby, 2007). The central tenet of the approach is that work (employment) is seen as an economic good, providing positive benefits for the individual, state and society. Yet little attention is paid to either the individual or the quality of that work. Indeed, the title of a UK government paper introducing the Flexible New Deal implemented from October 2009 (Cm 7130) and published in July 2007 was *In work – better off*. Above all this, there is the clearest indication of an individualistic approach to health in the Black report (2008). Here it states: 'Individuals have a fundamental personal responsibility for maintaining their own health' (Black, 2008, p 109). Accordingly, it is your own fault if you fall ill, not the result of, say, an industrial injury. Social factors appear to be secondary when set beside the activity and influence of individuals themselves.

Discussion

This chapter has suggested that the HWWB report was high on positive rhetoric for a workplace-based solution and yet when the strategy was implemented, it has been dominated by a medical model of health, with little recognition of the importance of preventative strategies within a workplace setting. More positively, it did place the issue of the benefits of better quality work and individual health and wellbeing higher up the policy agenda. However, it failed to look to other well-documented, thoroughly researched and supported approaches, and in particular those adopted by Finland and the subject of this chapter. This begs the question of why this successful approach was ignored and what might be the barriers to the successful implementation of a Work Ability approach.

So, the final part of this chapter will attempt to offer a case for adoption of a Work Ability approach to the UK. The effects of poor health and illness on the UK economy have already been cited and Black (2008) suggested that the costs of working-age ill health to the UK economy were in the region of £103 billion to £129 billion (Black 2008, p 46). That there is a compelling social and economic case to improve the health and wellbeing of the population is almost universally agreed. Within Black (2008), there are some useful case-study examples of forward-looking employers who see the benefits of better workplace health and wellbeing, even if this is often from a business-case perspective. However, many of these examples of good practice (documented on the HWWB website; see HWWB, 2010) tackle single issues (for example, smoking cessation, 'healthy' eating) that are not integrated into a holistic approach and therefore are of limited impact. Such strategies are also often unmonitored or scientifically assessed as to their impact on the health and wellbeing of individual employees, so remain tokenistic. A Work Ability approach would effectively tackle all these issues.

More positively, Black (2008) does mention a literature review conducted by the Peninsula Medical School (Campbell et al, 2007) that argues that early intervention can only be effective when a biopsychosocial model is adopted; that tailored services are delivered to the 'needs of the patient' and that 'case managers help with navigation and facilitate communication' (Black, 2008, pp 75-6). Although this argument has some positive features, there is an assumption here that *intervention* is preferable to a *preventative* strategy and that individuals are treated as *patients* primarily within a clinical setting. This is in contrast to the Work Ability approach, which is preventative, incorporates a scientifically derived measure and provides guidance on a range of interventions that when adopted benefit not only the individual but also the enterprise and often take place at the workplace.

Confusingly, even though these arguments might be seen as a step forward, it was later argued in Black (2008, p 76) that the evidence for the cited approach by the Peninsula Medical School was narrow (as it was based primarily on back pain) and such strategies could only work in countries 'outside Britain' (that is, Finland, Denmark, Canada and the Netherlands) because they had more comprehensive occupational health support than the UK. That point may be true but can be overcome. Indeed, Black (2008) incongruously devotes a whole chapter to a call for closer integration of the occupational health services within the National Health Service in the UK (Black, 2008, chapter 10). Nevertheless, an enhanced occupational health service and delivery is to be warmly welcomed as long overdue.

However, over and above this, it is clear that Black's (2008) report and recommendations can be seen as a wasted opportunity and is limited in its application. The focus on the fit-for-work process allows the medical profession to retain much of the delivery of the UK approach to workplace health and wellbeing within a clinical setting and model. Black (2008) ignores the substantial body of evidence on a Work Ability approach from Finland (and elsewhere) on flimsy grounds and seems to wish to 'reinvent the wheel'. The fit-for-work measures are simply an extension of the 'work first'/'work as welfare' ideology of the previous administration, driving people with medical conditions back into work as part of the desire to reduce the numbers on Employment Support Allowance. The Fit for Work programme is consequently in reality a sickness management strategy, not a programme to enhance the health and wellbeing of individuals.

Conclusion

A major argument of this chapter is that improving the health and wellbeing of adults must be seen as the public duty of government. This in effect means the promotion of better-quality working lives, the full expression of the 'active ageing' principle (Walker, 2002; WHO, 2002), applying it to working time as well as non-working time across the life-course. One means of achieving this is through the Work Ability approach discussed here. In this light, it is further suggested that the government allocate research funding to pilot the Work Ability approach, on a voluntary basis at first, across the UK, prior to its full implementation, producing publicity materials and incentives (financial or otherwise) to encourage employer take-up. Indeed, there is historical precedent for similar proactive governmental measures to improve the health and wellbeing and quality of work over the years, often supported by statute (such as pensions, working hours, factory work conditions, health and safety legislation and so on).

Following Lindley et al (2006), it seems that it is not a lack of knowledge on how to measure improved workplace health and wellbeing, nor implement a Work Ability approach, that is absent. Rather, it is engendering the desire and ability to bridge what Pfeffer and Sutton (2000) describe as the 'knowing-doing' gap, or the gap between knowledge and action. This is where we stand at present and why business, government and the research community must support longitudinal pilot investigations across the UK in a variety of businesses and sectors prior to a full implementation of work ability-based methods within enterprises.

Note
[1] Bilk Op Werk website (www.bilkopwerk.nl).

Further reading
Lindley, R. and Duell, N., with Arnkil, R., Baldauf, B., Bosworth, D., Casey, B., Gelderblom, A. and Leitzke, S. (2006) *Ageing and employment: Identification of good practice to increase job opportunities and maintain older workers in employment. Final report*, Brussels: European Commission, Directorate-General for Employment Social Affairs and Equal Opportunities.

Gould, R., Ilmarinen, J., Järvisalo J. and Koskinen S. (eds) (2008) *Dimensions of Work Ability. Results of the Health 2000 Survey*, Helsinki: Finnish Centre for Pensions, Social Insurance Institution, National Public Health Institute and Finnish Institute of Occupational Health.

Ilmarinen, J. (2005) *Towards a longer worklife! Ageing and the quality of worklife in the European Union*, Helsinki: Finnish Institute of Occupational Health, Ministry of Social Affairs and Health.

ILO (International Labour Organization) (2006) *Changing patterns in the world of work. Report of the Director General*, Geneva: ILO.

Maltby, T. (2010) ' "Older workers", workplace training and better quality working lives. Can a Workability approach help?', *International Journal of Education and Ageing*, vol 1, no 2, pp 141-52.

References

Black, C. (2008) *Working for a healthier tomorrow*, London: The Stationery Office.

Borrell-Carrió, F., Suchman, A.L. and Epstein, R.M. (2004) 'The biopsychosocial model 25 years later: principles, practice, and scientific inquiry', *Annals of Family Medicine,* vol 2, pp 576-82.

Campbell, J., Wright, C., Moseley, A., Chilvers, R., Richards, S. and Stabb, L. (2007) *Avoiding long-term incapacity for work: Developing an early intervention in primary care. A report of scoping work carried out by the Peninsula Medical School, Primary Care Research Group, on behalf of the Department for Work and Pensions (Health Work and Wellbeing)*, Exeter and Plymouth: Peninsula Medical School, Universities of Exeter and Plymouth.

Dini, E. (2009) 'Older workers in the UK: variations in economic activity status by socio-demographic characteristics, household and caring commitments', *Population Trends*, vol 137, Autumn, pp 11-24.

DSS (Department of Social Security) (1998) *New ambitions for our country: A new contract for welfare*, Cm 3805, London: The Stationery Office.

Engel, G.L. (1977) 'The need for a new medical model: a challenge for biomedicine', *Science*, vol 196, no 4286, pp 129-36.

Gould, R., Ilmarinen, J., Järvisalo, J. and Koskinen, S. (eds) (2008) *Dimensions of Work Ability. Results of the Health 2000 Survey*, Helsinki: Finnish Centre for Pensions, Social Insurance Institution, National Public Health Institute and Finnish Institute of Occupational Health.

Griffiths, A. (2007) 'Healthy work for older workers: work design and management factors', in W. Loretto, S. Vickerstaff and P. White (eds) *The future for older workers: New perspectives*, Bristol: The Policy Press, pp 121-38.

Hill, D., Lucy, D., Tyers, C. and James L. (2007) *What works at work?*, Leeds: The Stationery Office.

Humphrey, A., Costigan, P., Pickering, K., Stratford, N. and Barnes, M. (2003) *Factors affecting the labour market participation of older workers*, DWP Research Report 200, London: Department for Work and Pensions.

HSE (Health and Safety Executive) (2010) HSE Health, Work and Well-being website, www.hse.gov.uk/hwwb

HWWB (Health, Work and Wellbeing) (2010) HWWB website, www.dwp.gov.uk/health-work-and-well-being

Ilmarinen, J. (ed) (1991) 'The aging worker', *Scandinavian Journal of Work Environment and Health*, vol 17, no 1. Supplement 1.

Ilmarinen, J. (1999) *Ageing workers in the European Union. Status and promotion of work ability, employability and employment*, Helsinki: Finnish Institute of Occupational Health, Ministry of Social Affairs and Health Ministry of Labour.

Ilmarinen, J. (2005) *Towards a longer worklife! Ageing and the quality of worklife in the European Union*, Helsinki: Finnish Institute of Occupational Health, Ministry of Social Affairs and Health.

Ilmarinen, J. (2010) '30 years of Work Ability and 20 years of age management in Finland', Paper presented to 4th Symposium on Work Ability, Tampere, Finland, June.

Ilmarinen, J. and Tuomi, K. (2004) 'Past, present and future of work ability', *People and Work Research Reports*, vol 65, pp 1-25.

Ilmarinen, J., Tuomi, K., Eskelinen, L., Nygård, C.-H., Huuhtanen, P. and Klockars, M. (1991) 'Background and objectives of the Finnish research project on aging workers in municipal occupations', *Scandinavian Journal of Environmental Health*, vol 17, Supplement 1, pp 7-11.

ILO (International Labour Organisation) (2006) *Changing patterns in the world of work. Report of the Director General*, Geneva: ILO.

Irving, P., Steels, J. and Hall, N. (2005) *Factors affecting the labour market participation of older workers: Qualitative research*, DWP Research Report 281, London: Department for Work and Pensions.

Lindley, R. and Duell, N., with Arnkil, R., Baldauf, B., Bosworth, D., Casey, B., Gelderblom, A. and Leitzke, S. (2006) *Ageing and employment: Identification of good practice to increase job opportunities and maintain older workers in employment. Final report*, Brussels: European Commission, Directorate-General for Employment Social Affairs and Equal Opportunities.

Maltby, T. (2007) 'The employability of "older workers": what works', in W. Loretto, S. Vickerstaff and P. White (eds) *The future for older workers: New perspectives*, Bristol: The Policy Press, pp 161-84.

Maltby, T. (2011) 'Extending working lives? Employability, work ability and better quality working lives', *Social Policy and Society*, vol 10, no 3, pp 299-308.

McNair, S. and Flynn, M. (2006) *Older workers in the South East*, Guildford: Centre for Research on Older Workers (CROW).

Navarro, V. (1978) *Class struggle, the state and medicine: An historical and contemporary analysis of the medical sector in Great Britain*, London: Martin Robertson.

OASPG (Opportunity Age Strategy Policy Group) (2008) *Summary of work of the Health, Work and Well-being Strategy (HWWB)*, Opportunity Age Strategy Policy Group, Employment Sub Group Briefing Paper, February [Unpublished].

ONS (2009) *Statistical Bulletin Older People's Day 2009*, London: TSO.

Peltomäki, P., Husman, K. and Vertio, H. (2002) 'The process and maintenance of work ability in Finnish workplaces. What do we know about the prerequisites of a successful MWA', in P. Peltomäki, K. Husman and H. Vertio (eds) *Maintainence of work ability and assessment: Summaries report 7*, Helsinki: Ministry of Social Affairs and Health, Finnish Institute of Occupational Health and Social Insurance Institution of Finland, pp 17-21.

Pfeffer, J. and Sutton, R.I. (2000) 'The knowing–doing gap', in *Public in the age of uncertainty*, Cambridge: Polity Press, pp 23-40.

Phillipson, C. and Smith, A. (2005) *Extending working life: A review of the research literature*, DWP Research Report 299, London: Department for Work and Pensions.

Smeaton, D. and Vegeris, S. (2009) *Older workers inside and outside the labour market: A review*, EHRC Research Report 22, Manchester: Equalities and Human Rights Commission.

Smeaton, D., Vegeris, S. and Sahin-Dimen, M. (2008) *Older workers: Employment preferences, barriers and solutions*, EHRC Research Report 43, Manchester: Equalities and Human Rights Commission.

Rose, G., with Khaw, K.-T. and Marmot, M. (2008) *The strategy of preventative medicine*, Oxford: Oxford University Press.

Taylor, P., Mclaughlin, C., Oakman, J., Palermo, J., Parker, T., Worringham, C. and Swan, P. (2010) 'Workability measurement in Australia: A Work Ability Index databank', Paper presented to 4th Symposium on Work Ability, Tampere, Finland, June.

Townsend, P. and Davidson, N. (1981) *Inequalities in health, the Black report*, Harmondsworth: Penguin.

Tuomi, K. (ed) (1997) 'Eleven year follow-up of aging workers', *Scandinavian Journal of Environmental Health*, vol 23, Supplement 1.

Tuomi, K., Huuhtanen, P., Nykyri, E. and Ilmarinen, J. (2001) 'Promotion of work ability, the quality of work and retirement', *Occupational Medicine*, vol 51, no 5, pp 318-24.

Tuomi, K., Ilmarinen, J., Eskelinen, L., Järvinen, E., Toikkanen, J., and Klocklars, M. (1991) 'Prevalence and incidence rates of diseases and workability in different work categories', *Scandinavian Journal of Environmental Health*, vol 17, no 1, pp 67-74.

Tuomi, K., Ilmarinen, J., Jahkola, A., Katajarinne, L. and Tulkki, A. (1998) *Work Ability Index*, Helsinki: Finnish Institute of Occupational Health.

Tuomi, K., Wägar, G., Eskelinen, L., Järvinen, E., Huuhtanen, P., Suurnäkki, T., Fahlström, P., Aalto, L. and Ilmarinen, J. (1985) 'Health work capacity and work conditions in municipal occupations', *Työterveyslaitoksen* tutkimuksia, vol 3, no 2, pp 95-132 [in Finnish with English abstract].

Vickerstaff, S., Loretto, W., Billings, J., Brown, P., Mitton, L., Parkin, T. and White, P. (2008) *Encouraging labour market activity among 60-64 year olds*, DWP Research Report No 531, London: Department for Work and Pensions.

Waddell, G. and Burton, A.K. (2006) *Is work good for your health and wellbeing?*, London: The Stationery Office.

Walker, A., (2002) 'A strategy for active ageing', *International Social Security Review*, vol 55, no 1, pp 121-39.

WHO (World Health Organization) (2002) *Active ageing: A policy framework*, Geneva: WHO.

ELEVEN

Working for longer: self-management of chronic health problems in the workplace

Fehmidah Munir

Introduction

This chapter considers how employees with health problems can maintain their own health, wellbeing and productivity across over their working life. Chronic health problems are an increasing problem within an ageing workforce. The majority of these health issues are defined as a *'condition that is long-term, cannot be* currently cured but can be controlled with the use of medication and/or other therapies' (DH, 2010, p 4). Such conditions can be limiting in terms of daily functioning. They include common health problems such as musculoskeletal disorders (such as repetitive strain injury and persistent back pain) and mental health problems (such as stress, anxiety and depression), as well as cardio-respiratory conditions. Although health issues are generally associated with an ageing population, many conditions are caused, or made worse, by work (HSE, 2010). Musculoskeletal disorders and stress, depression or anxiety are the most commonly reported work-related health problems. They are also reported to be the biggest causes of both long-term and short-term sick leave (CIPD, 2009) and the most common reason for claiming incapacity benefits (HSE, 2008).

The prevalence of chronic health problems at work is potentially higher when those with a non-work-related but *work-relevant* health problem are included in the figures (that is, causes of disability, absenteeism and work loss). Common examples include HIV, rheumatoid arthritis, diabetes and cancer. Despite this, the prevalence of people with a chronic health problem in employment in the UK is much lower compared with rates from counterpart countries: approximately 59% of British men compared with over 70% of their Danish and Norwegian counterparts; and half of British women compared with over 64% of their Norwegian and Swedish counterparts (Whitehead et al, 2009).

Overall, the annual costs of sickness absences and unemployment related to chronic health problems is over £100 billion, equivalent to the annual costs of the National Health Service (Black, 2008). It is widely acknowledged that work is good for health and can reduce health inequalities (Waddell and Burton, 2006). Furthermore, job retention or (return to) work is therapeutic for most people with health problems, as it promotes recovery and rehabilitation, and maintains or improves quality of life and wellbeing (Waddell and Burton, 2006). There are therefore benefits to society as a whole in keeping employees healthy and productive at work.

Both EU and UK policymakers have identified key strategies to address the impact of work-relevant chronic health problems on healthcare and social care expenditure (Curtis, 2003; Black, 2008). In the, these include:

- facilitating the employability of people with chronic health problems;
- reducing the number of working days lost due to work-related injury and ill health;
- supporting businesses to appreciate the cost benefits of investing in employee health and wellbeing;
- encouraging good occupational health services provision;
- promoting public health initiatives in the workplace such as tackling stress and obesity;
- developing services to help people return to, or remain in work;
- incorporating work-related outcomes into future national public health guidelines (DETR, 2000; DWP, 2008).

A key theme running through these strategies is the recognition of the links between health, wellbeing and behaviour. A strong emphasis is also placed on early intervention from a biopsychosocial perspective. This model simultaneously considers the interplay between biological (for example, disease or condition), psychological (for example, coping strategies), social (for example, social support, organisational culture) and macro (for example, policies) levels (Lunt et al, 2007). It recognises that most chronic health problems are associated with biological and behavioural risk factors, and that social and cultural factors play a significant role in how illness is experienced by the affected person (WHO, 2008a). Current government initiatives do address some of the clinical, social and economic aspects in effectively managing chronic health problems in the workplace. Improving employee 'self-management' behaviours is less explicit, but nevertheless underpinned by some of these initiatives.

So what is self-management, why is it important and how do current initiatives address it? This chapter first outlines what self-management is, its importance to individuals with a chronic health problem and current healthcare interventions to support self-management activities. Next, it reviews the evidence for work and health outcomes associated with good self-management behaviours in the workplace, and discusses current workplace interventions and new directions that enhance self-management behaviours and skills.

Self-management: definitions, concepts and behaviours

Self-management broadly refers to a set of actions undertaken by an individual to manage his or her chronic health problem on a day-to-day basis. These actions are considered different from those undertaken by a 'healthy' individual as a preventative strategy to ill health (Clark et al, 1991). Several definitions and concepts exist to encapsulate self-management. According to Corbin and Strauss (1988), self-management consists of three tasks:

- medication or behavioural management (such as adhering to a special diet);
- role management (such as adjusting previous roles or tasks to accommodate the illness); and
- emotional management (managing anger, fear, frustration or low mood experienced as a result of having a chronic health problem).

These tasks are based around the shifting perspectives of the individual and their perceived problems. Corbin and Strauss's framework therefore acknowledges that some illnesses (or illness symptoms) are episodic and may vary in terms of severity, therefore requiring different self-management tasks as appropriate. Other definitions incorporate psychological and social management much more centrally. For example, Clark et al (1991) and Gallant (2003) view self-management as a host of activities that include not only recognising and responding to symptoms, managing acute episodes and use of medication; but also managing relations and obtaining support from significant others. They suggest that self-management is influenced by contextual factors such as social networks, family support, healthcare provision, and the physical environment. Similarly, Barlow and colleagues (2002) regard self-management as the individual's ability to manage their condition through cognitive, behavioural and emotional responses required to sustain a satisfactory quality of life. This definition also includes an individual's ability to manage the physical and psychosocial consequences and lifestyle changes associated with a chronic health problem. Barlow and colleagues therefore view self-management as a dynamic and continuous process of self-regulation (Barlow, 2001).

The importance of self-management for chronic health problems has led to a number of health policies in the UK and elsewhere, such as the US and Australia (DH, 1999, 2010; Center for the Advancement of Health, 2002; Glasgow et al, 2008). The policies outline provisions for case management for complex conditions, disease management for conditions with medium long-term risk of complications, and self-management programmes for low-risk, long-term health conditions. In the UK, the Expert Patients Programme delivers self-management support and skills to help individuals take more effective control over their illness and quality of life (DH, 2001). The main aim of self-management programmes is to facilitate behaviours such as appropriate diet, exercise, medication use, symptom management and pain management by empowering individuals to define their goals, take responsibility for their treatment and increase their autonomy (Feste and Anderson, 1995; Varekamp et al, 2009). This is achieved by increasing individuals' confidence and motivation, and developing communication, problem-solving and action-planning skills by utilising appropriate psychological theory.

One of the key theories used in self-management programmes is self-efficacy (Bandura, 1977), defined as 'belief in one's capabilities to organize and execute the courses of action required to produce given attainments' (Bandura, 1997, p 3). Self-efficacy beliefs operate along with goals in the regulation of motivation, behaviour and wellbeing (Bandura, 1997), and are measured by assessing one's belief or confidence to achieve a goal, for example successfully managing pain associated with a particular health condition. Self-management intervention studies have shown that changes to self-efficacy are associated with changes in behaviour and health status for a range of chronic health issues such as arthritis, cardiovascular conditions, respiratory conditions and diabetes (for example, Lorig et al, 2001; Griffiths et al, 2005; Reeves et al, 2008). Other theories utilised in self-management programmes include cognitive behavioural therapy (CBT), which aims to change how people think about their chronic health problem and how their thoughts feed into behaviour (Michie and Abraham, 2004). Self-management programmes utilising this theory have been particularly beneficial for mental health problems (Layard,

2005) as well as musculoskeletal problems such as persistent back pain (Moore et al, 2000).

The effectiveness of self-management programmes has been reported in a number of review studies (Barlow et al, 2002; Newman et al, 2004; Plack et al, 2010). Overall, there is good evidence that, when compared with standard care, self-management programmes provide benefits in performance of health behaviours and health outcomes (Barlow et al, 2002). For example, arthritis self-management programmes report improvements in pain and physical functioning as well as in exercise, self-efficacy and positive wellbeing (Barlow et al, 2000). Asthma self-management programmes have reduced hospitalisations, emergency room visits and nocturnal asthma (Gibson et al, 2002), and diabetes programmes demonstrate increases in self-management behaviours such as blood glucose monitoring and subsequent reductions in glycated haemoglobin (Plack et al, 2010). Self-management programmes for chronic heart failure also demonstrate some improvement in quality of life and reduced hospital admissions (Ditewig et al, 2010).

Despite the benefits of self-management programmes in terms of changes in behaviour, health status and wellbeing, the effectiveness of these programmes is considered to be small in some cases. One of the main obstacles to self-management is low adherence to carrying out self-management activities by individuals. Factors attributed to low adherence include lack of acceptance of the chronic health problem, poor psychological adjustment, co-morbidity of depression, and finding self-management a burden and having difficulty integrating it into daily life (see DeRidder et al, 2008, for a review). Self-management programmes are mainly standalone and do not take into account the wider social context of the individual with a chronic health problem, such as the social and material resources available to them, and whether they are employed or claiming benefits, their type of employment (for example, manual work), as well as the role played by these wider social contexts in the individual's self-management of their chronic health. Furthermore, numerous socio-political, community and cultural factors interact to influence health outcomes in those with a chronic health problem (Whittemore and Dixon, 2008). It is now proposed that self-management interventions should be optimised by taking a more complete biopsychosocial approach in the delivery of such programmes, whether are lay or expert-led (Glasgow et al, 2008; Rogers et al, 2008; Rogers, 2009). Glasgow and colleagues (2008) argue that there should be increased efforts to integrate self-management support activities with other sectors such as the workplace. This is also suggested by Wesson and Gould (2010) and by Rogers (2009).

Given that chronic health problems such as rheumatoid arthritis, asthma, chronic obstructive pulmonary disease (COPD) and diabetes are predicted to increase in the working population over the next 20 years (Blokstra et al, 2007; Bhattacharya et al, 2008), integrating self-management intervention programmes with current workplace initiatives makes good sense. Before integrating self-management programmes into the workplace, an understanding is required of how employees currently manage their chronic health problem within the workplace, which psychosocial and workplace factors influence their ability to manage their health and what they need in order to effectively manage both their chronic health problem and their work demands. The current evidence for this is reviewed in the next section.

Self-management of behaviours in the workplace

It is well documented that a significant number of employees with a chronic health problem report experiencing difficulties in meeting physical and/or psychosocial work demands of their job (Lerner, et al, 2000; Munir et al, 2005a; Roelen et al, 2008) and are at risk of work disability (Detaille et al, 2009). This includes those with diabetes, cardiovascular disease (Burton et al, 1999), hypertension, arthritis, asthma (Kessler et al, 2003), cancer and depression (Kessler et al, 2001), who report not only work impairments but also higher sickness absence compared with those without a chronic health problem (Roskes et al, 2005; Munir et al, 2008). Those with depression report greater impairments on psychosocial work demands compared with other chronic health problems (Burton et al, 2004). However, those with cancer report the greatest impairment on both physical and psychosocial work demands (Kessler et al, 2001; Munir et al, 2009a). Work limitations increase with increasing co-morbidity (that is, more than one chronic health problem) (Lerner et al, 2000; Kessler et al, 2001, 2003). Co-morbidity is also linked with more sickness absence (Kessler et al, 2003).

Despite these problems, evidence suggests that many individuals with a chronic health problem want to remain in active employment (Mancuso et al, 2000). Several studies have documented the obstacles and facilitators to this, including:

- the health problem itself (Lerner et al, 2000; Kessler et al, 2001);
- the socioeconomic context (Waddell and Aylward, 2005; Barnes et al, 2008);
- work characteristics and workplace support (Munir et al, 2005a);

- organisational policies and procedures and organisational culture (Kopina and Haafkens, 2009).

Less attention has been paid to how employees' perceptions and behaviour towards their chronic health problem and work could be targeted by intervention to improve health and employment outcomes. This is an important area for both research and intervention, as it is suggested that those who have their chronic health problem under control through good self-management are more likely to remain active in employment for longer, that is, the healthy worker effect (Munir et al, 2009b). In contrast those who have poor self-management skills are more likely to either exit from the workforce or take early ill-health retirement (Munnell and Libby, 2007). Studies that have examined self-management behaviours among employees with a chronic health problem have focused on a biopsychosocial perspective by considering the workplace context and the impact it has on health, wellbeing and productivity. Munir et al (2005b, 2008, 2009b) examined health behaviours carried out in the workplace such as taking medication, managing symptoms, exercising, disclosing illness and making a adjustments to their work. These behaviours were examined among employees with a range of chronic health problems. They found that most employees carried out key self-management behaviours in the workplace as well as outside the workplace. These included taking medication, managing symptoms, seeking support from colleagues and making adjustments to their work (Munir et al, 2005b). They also found that although some employees were forced to disclose their illness to their employers due to sickness absence (Munir et al, 2008), most chose to disclose their illness to their line managers to access support and work adjustments (Munir et al, 2005c).

Although disclosure of a chronic health problem does not always result in workplace changes for all chronic health problems, especially depression (Munir 2005a; Gignac and Cao, 2009), facilitative changes in work arrangements do occur for a significant number of employees who disclose their illness. These include reduced working hours and adjustments to the physical working environment (Lerner et al, 2000; Baanders et al, 2001). Workplace changes are therefore crucial to employees in managing their chronic health problem and their work productivity. In a study by Gignac et al (2002) employees with arthritis had better health outcomes at work such as reduced symptoms and increased psychological well-being, if they were able to make at least one workplace adjustment to manage their chronic health problem at work (Gignac et al 2002).

The findings from these studies suggest that good self-management behaviours could reduce not only sickness absence but also sickness presenteeism (that is, turning up for work despite feeling ill). However, this can only be achieved if employees are given control over their working environment to make the changes they need in order to manage both their chronic health problem and their work. In addition, organisational factors such as attendance policies and procedures (Munir et al, 2008; Wynne-Jones et al, 2010), constrained working-time arrangements (Böckerman and Laukkanen, 2009), poor work characteristics (Varekamp and van Dijk, 2010) and the illness perceptions of line managers (Munir et al, 2005a; Wynne-Jones et al, 2010) can also affect how successfully employees are able to carry out self-management behaviours at work. These factors are complex and further reinforce the need for a biopsychosocial approach to managing the impact of chronic health problems on the health and work status of employees.

A small number of studies have examined the psychological factors that determine self-management behaviours in the workplace. Weijman et al (2005) found that employees with diabetes with high self-efficacy were able to manage their condition in the workplace, and their workload and work pressures, more effectively. In contrast, those with low self-efficacy and those with an avoidance coping style perceived self-management behaviours at work as a burden. Lack of self-acceptance of having a chronic health problem also created obstacles to self-management behaviours (Varekamp and van Dijk, 2010). Detaille et al (2003) and Gignac (2005) found that coping with a chronic health problem at work was an important determinant for both health and work outcomes. Munir et al (2009c) reported that employees who had high self-efficacy in taking medication, managing symptoms and making changes to their work, were more likely to carry out these behaviours at work. Furthermore, they found that line manager support was directly related to these self-management behaviours, and also positively influenced employees' self-efficacy.

The importance of receiving support for self-management behaviours is well documented in the health literature (for example, Gallant, 2003). Equally, the importance of line manager support for health and wellbeing is well documented in the occupational literature. Line manager support has been related to better work adjustments (Munir et al, 2005a) and improved stressor–strain relationships and job performance (de Lange et al, 2003; Stetz et al, 2006), and has also been associated with reducing symptoms of depression among employees over time (Munir et al, 2010). Seeking support is therefore an important contextual self-management behaviour that has positive outcomes on the health and work status of those employees with a chronic health problem. Not receiving the required support that is appropriate both in the practical and empathic sense may have negative consequences on employee health status and can result in sickness presenteeism, sickness absenteeism, delayed return to work or exit from the workforce (Michie and Williams, 2003). This is especially important for those with musculoskeletal disorders who are faced with a number of barriers and obstacles in returning to, or maintaining, work (Waddell and Burton, 2006), and for those with depression who have poor coping, low self-efficacy and low self-management skills compared with other illness groups (DeRidder et al, 2008; Munir et al, 2009b). However, the nature of these health problems is further complicated by the contribution of work factors to the illness itself. It is therefore not surprising that most research on psychosocial factors relating to causes of sickness absence and return to work have focused on these two common health problems.

Much attention has been paid to the working conditions and organisational systems and policies that contribute to ill health, sickness absence and length of sick leave for those with musculoskeletal disorders (Main et al, 2007) and those with stress, depression and anxiety (Michie and Williams, 2003). Equally, attention has been paid to individual factors (such as age and educational level) that contribute to sickness absence and return to work. Although the concept of self-management as a determinant of sickness absence and return to work has not been considered explicitly, the psychological and behavioural factors that play a role in general self-management behaviours have been reported as playing a role in sickness absence and return-to-work outcomes. For persistent back pain, co-morbidity of depression, high and persistent pain levels, poorer self-reported health status and functional limitations, poor expectations of recovery, and fear that undertaking activities will aggravate the problem, have been associated with sickness absence and low return-to-work outcomes (Linton and Halldén, 1998; Currie and Wang, 2004; Kuijer et al, 2006; Meijer et al, 2006; Dionne et al, 2007). For those with anxiety and depression, fear of relapse, fear of exposure to the initial scenario that caused the illness and severity of the illness have also been associated with low return-to-work outcomes (Baanders et al, 2001; Nieuwenhuijsen et al, 2003). A few studies have also examined the psychological and behavioural factors that affect return-to-work outcomes among those with cardiovascular conditions. Emotional problems, distress, depression, anxiety, misconceptions about health, preoccupation with symptoms and lack of social support are reported to affect return-to-work outcomes (Waddell and Burton, 2006). Similarly, depression and anxiety affect return-to-work outcomes among those recovering from cancer. Treatment side-effects, such as fatigue, cognitive problems, poor sleep and lack of support, also affect work ability (Taskila and Lindbohm, 2007; Munir et al, 2009a).

The evidence from these studies suggest that work-related interventions are required that address the psychological factors, shift behavioural attitudes and deliver self-management skills among those with a chronic health problem so that these individuals can effectively manage their chronic health problem and their work. Such interventions do exist and are now widespread across many organisations, occupational health services and rehabilitation services. However, they predominantly focus on either prevention of certain chronic health problems or on interventions that aid return to work and are therefore more or less focused on rehabilitation. Employees with non-work-related health problems who do not fall under a legislative Act such as the 2010 Equality Act in the UK, are often overlooked in interventions. These employees may not have taken long-term sick leave but are at risk in doing so further down the line if self-management of their chronic health problem becomes burdensome, complex or difficult to carry out due to workplace obstacles and difficulties in making workplace adjustments. There are many workplace health management initiatives and workplace policies that can easily be adapted to include or integrate self-management programmes, whether these are led by in-house occupational health professionals or bought-in services. Following on is a review of current interventions where elements of self-management support and training are evident, although not necessarily labelled as self-management interventions.

Workplace interventions that enhance self-management behaviours and skills

Workplace interventions for chronic health problems generally fall into three broad types:

* prevention (such as health promotion activities);
* management of health problems as they arise (secondary prevention); and
* and rehabilitation (such as managing long-term sickness absence and return to work).

Workplace health promotion programmes are initiatives designed to improve the health and wellbeing of employees. These include activities such as promoting increased physical activity, smoking cessation and healthy eating. They are usually targeted at both the healthy working population and those at risk of a developing a health problem such as cardiovascular disease, diabetes and obesity. Interventions range from education-based programmes and individually tailored risk-reduction counselling to multimethod approaches targeted at both individual behaviour change and changes at the organisational level (for example, introducing flexible working conditions, modifying the work environment) (Goetzel et al, 2008). A number of workplace health promotion programmes also utilise appropriate theory such self-efficacy and CBT that enable employees to develop goals and objectives in achieving behaviour change (Goetzel et al, 2008).

There is good evidence that general health promotion programmes such as physical activity and initiatives targeted at lifestyle change are effective in improving health (such as fitness), wellbeing and work ability; and in reducing sickness absence (Kuoppala et al, 2008; Abraham and Graham-Rowe, 2009). Specific health promotion programmes that are targeted at reducing risk factors for cardiovascular disease (such as improving diet) or depression and anxiety symptoms (for example, skills training, stress management) are also reported to be quite effective (Seymour and Grove, 2005; Martin et al, 2009; Groeneveld et al, 2010). A number of health promotion initiatives are also targeted at preventing musculoskeletal disorders (such as back pain) using exercise, education, training and ergonomic interventions. These approaches have been reported to be moderately effective in preventing musculoskeletal problems (Maher, 2000; Gatty et al, 2003; Rivilis et al, 2008).

Unfortunately, the majority of workplace health promotion programmes do not report separate health outcomes and other indicators (such as sickness absence) for those already managing a chronic health problem other than musculoskeletal disorders and mental health problems. Furthermore, it is also not known to what extent the methods used in workplace health programmes (for example, counselling, group education, goal setting) help to improve and support the self-management skills and behaviours of those with a chronic health problem. There is a missed opportunity for both researchers and practitioners to tease out the effects of workplace health promotion initiatives for specific chronic health problems that are already prevalent in the workplace. One suggestion as to why this has not yet become a key focus of research or chronic health management initiatives is that although health promotion programmes can be beneficial to future health, this same assumption may not hold for people already managing a chronic health problem (Lorig and Laurin, 1985; Lorig and Holman, 2003). Workplace health promotion programmes do not take into account the complexity of factors that influence the health outcomes for those with a specific chronic health problem. These include the pathological changes that occur in some chronic health problems and that are non-reversible, and the sociological and cultural factors and other important mediators such as the healthcare system and significant others (for example, partners) that play a role in the management of chronic health problems (Glasgow and Eakin, 1998; Whittemore and Dixon, 2008). For these reasons, workplace interventions have largely focused on lifestyle factors that may lead to future chronic health problems they can control indirectly, or only those chronic health problems that they can control more directly, such as work-related chronic health problems, that is, mental health problems, cardio-respiratory conditions and musculoskeletal disorders (Hassan, et al, 2009).

Not surprisingly, there is extensive literature on the management (secondary prevention) and rehabilitation of employees with health problems such as stress, back pain and cardiovascular conditions (see Waddell and Burton, 2006, Hill et al, 2007; Hassan et al, 2009 for an extensive review of these). These take a biopsychosocial approach, particularly for musculoskeletal disorders such as persistent back pain. Interventions for the latter often include addressing a number of specific factors such as health condition (healthcare), personal and/or psychological factors, organisational and systems obstacles, psychosocial aspects of work and attitudes to health and disability (Waddell and Burton, 2004). Some of these interventions directly and indirectly target self-management behaviours and skills, particularly with regard to pain management, as means of reducing length of work disability and sickness absence (Waddell and Burton, 2001; Franche et al, 2005; Hill et al, 2007; Hassan et al, 2009). These range from providing informational advice about staying active to cognitive behavioural interventions addressing attitudes and behaviours such as fear of movement and teaching problem-solving skills to reduce sickness absence, improve return-to-work outcomes and reduce work disability. Moreover, there is strong evidence for an integrated approach in reducing work disability that includes work accommodation and contact between healthcare provider and the workplace in managing and rehabilitating those with musculoskeletal disorders (Franche et al, 2005).

Interventions for managing and rehabilitating those with mental health problems can be categorised into organisational-level interventions, which consist of job reorganisation, supervisory training and other education or cognitive initiatives, and individual-level interventions, which include CBT and other types of cognitive and educational interventions (Seymour and Grove, 2005). It is largely the latter category where some of the self-management behaviours and skills may be targeted, mostly through CBT. These include training in coping skills, personal support, action planning and goal setting (Seymour and Grove, 2005; Hassan et al, 2009). There is strong evidence that these types of intervention are very effective in reducing not only symptoms of psychological ill health, but also absenteeism (Seymour and Grove, 2005; Hill, 2007; Hassan et al, 2009).

A small number of work-related interventions have focused on cardio-respiratory conditions where similar interventions to those with musculoskeletal disorders and mental health problems are offered, targeting some self-management behaviours and skills (Waddell and Burton, 2006). Few of these interventions are extended to other chronic health problems. For most other types of chronic health problem, management in the workplace has largely been limited to disability management, offering work adjustments and work accommodations. However, the burden of a chronic health problem requires more than work adjustments, as chronic health conditions can be complex and challenging. Employees need help and support with the impact their condition may have on them emotionally; with adjusting to a life working with a chronic health problem; and with regaining wellness. Moreover, such employees require support in maintaining work participation that includes maintaining and extending meaningful roles and occupation at work, and maintaining relationships with significant others at work such as colleagues and line managers. This suggests the need for an expansion of current workplace models of managing ill health.

Workplace training in self-management skills and behaviours: new directions

There is now slow but growing recognition for the need to manage a wider range of chronic health problems in the workplace due to their increasing prevalence as the workforce ages and the impact they have on working life (Lerner et al, 2000; Munir et al, 2009b). In particular, the empowerment-oriented approach has been suggested as an effective way to enable employees not only to manage their chronic health problem, but also to maintain active employment (Varekamp et al, 2006).

According to Varekamp and colleagues (2009): 'In order for managers to implement appropriate accommodations it is necessary that employees understand their problems, discuss these with their supervisors and colleagues and reach a solution' (p 399). They designed a training programme for those with serious chronic health problem including rheumatic arthritis, Crohn's disease, COPD, cardiovascular heart disease and visual impairment. The programme addressed the following:

• practical and psychosocial obstacles and barriers to work quality;
• insights and thoughts about having a chronic health problem;
• communication at work;
• legalisation and facilities for disabled employees; and
• solving problems.

The training was delivered in group sessions that aimed to empower employees to define their work-related problems and potential solutions. Changes in perceived self-efficacy, job retention, fatigue and job satisfaction were the primary outcomes measures, with changes in sick leave, work-related problems and work accommodations as secondary outcome measures (Varekamp et al, 2008, 2009). The effectiveness of the intervention has not been reported prior to preparation of this book. So far, findings from the qualitative analysis of process change suggest the training has enabled employees to gain self-awareness of their abilities in relation to their chronic health problem, and to identify work-related problems and how to manage them. In support of this, there is some evidence that empowerment-based intervention programmes for employees with chronic health problems are effective in terms of skills and behaviour change for acquiring support and work accommodations, communication skills and increased self-confidence in managing with work-related problems (Allaire et al, 1996; Varekamp et al, 2006). However, most of these interventions have not directly addressed self-management of the chronic health problem itself, such as managing medication at work and monitoring symptoms. The primary focus is identifying and negotiating work-based solutions to maintain employment.

A more recent workplace intervention has adapted the Chronic Disease Self-Management Program (CDSMP) used in community and healthcare settings in the US. Detaille and colleagues (2010) used an intervention-mapping process (Bartholomew et al, 2006) to tailor the original programme for employees with a somatic chronic health problem. Based on the empowerment approach, they identified a self-management behaviour programme that would enable employees to ask for help and support from colleagues and supervisors; cope with symptoms such as pain, fatigue and emotional distress, and manage a healthy lifestyle; and manage work in relation to the chronic health problem. This would be achieved through behaviour change (such as changes in attitudes and beliefs), improving action–planning activity and increasing self-efficacy and self-regulatory capabilities. The strength of this particular intervention is that it is built to suit the needs of employees in different stages of behavioural change and with different behavioural goals, although it could be it difficult to evaluate the effectiveness of the intervention. As the intervention is relatively new, the results are not yet published.

There are a number of potential obstacles to implementing self-management programmes in the workplace that have not been fully considered by the above interventions.

First, many chronic health problems are invisible in terms of their symptoms not being apparent. Unless an employee is on sick leave, has a fit note from their GP or requires a legal workplace adjustment, they may not disclose their condition to their employer (Munir et al, 2008). This could potentially make it difficult to introduce workplace self-management interventions. Many chronic health problems are also highly stigmatised in the workplace, making disclosure even more difficult (Vickers, 1997; Munir et al, 2005c). Furthermore, those who disclose their chronic health problem have high self-efficacy and self-management skills and choose to disclose as part of their self-management strategy and access to support (Munir et al, 2005b). Therefore, those employees who are poorly managing their chronic health problem (regardless of severity), have not disclosed it and have not yet taken long-term sick leave are most likely in need of an integrated workplace self-management intervention.

Second, employees with a chronic health problem form an internally heterogeneous group (Kopina and Haafkens, 2010). Despite this, there are some common characteristics that can be targeted in a workplace self-management programme. Chronic health problems can be grouped into certain categories, for example those with constant symptoms and those that are episodic; those that are moderately stable and those that are progressive; and those that result in predominantly physical limitations and those that have predominantly mental limitations.

Third, many employers and human resource professionals are not always adequately trained to recognise chronic health problems. A review by Kopnina and Haafkens (2010) found that not only were most managers and human resource practitioners unaware of the impact of chronic health problems in their organisation and on an employee's working life, but also that most line managers do not have access to resources in order to implement European or national frameworks relating to workforce participation for those with a chronic health problem or disability. Organisations may have to take measures to change some aspects of the organisational culture that act as obstacles to effectively managing employees with chronic health problems, for example, introducing organisational procedures that may involve disclosure and reporting procedures to open dialogue between employees and their managers that may potentially lead to solutions (Kopnina and Haafkens, 2009).

The main concern regarding these new self-management interventions is that it is not yet known if they will be effective in a workplace setting. However, there is some evidence to suggest that a work-based self-management programme can be effective. Self-management training has been used to improve work attendance by training employees who have high sickness absence rates in self-regulatory skills to manage personal and social obstacles to attending work and to increase their self-efficacy in these skills (Frayne and Latham, 1987). Evidence from this intervention study suggests that self-management training in attendance is effective in increasing work attendance when compared with a control group (Frayne and Latham, 1987). Self-management training programmes have also been used to improve self-selected work-decisions and methods of work among work teams by training them to be autonomous in their work tasks. For example, training them to identify, monitor and implement an intervention for a work problem (Hackman 1987). The benefits for teams that self-manage their work are wide-ranging and include increased productivity and innovation, and also increased self-efficacy, support, wellbeing and job satisfaction (Manz and Sims, 1987; van Mierlo et al, 2005, 2007).

In general, the concept of 'self-management' and its benefits is not new to organisations. However, the challenge will be to shift not just the beliefs of employees and employers, but also those of occupational health professionals and other key stakeholders and policymakers about the importance of self-management programmes for chronic health problems in the workplace. Integrating self-management programmes into the workplace may not require substantial amounts of resources, but will require availability of appropriate services to support integration of self-management into the workplace. For example, there needs to be good communication between healthcare services, employers and employees themselves when healthcare services are delivering self-management programmes among individual employees. This is important for small and medium-sized enterprises that may not be able to deliver their own self-management programmes in conjunction with other services. For larger organisations with access to occupational health services, self-management programmes can be designed to complement and enhance healthcare-led self-management programmes. Except for medication management (which should be healthcare-led), most self-management skills are generic and many self-management programmes are holistic and multi-component. Therefore, workplaces can easily deliver self-management programmes to employees with a chronic health problem by following the same plan and system for workplace health promotion programmes.

Key elements of successful workplace health promotion programmes include:

- establishing clear goals and objectives, linking programmes to business objectives;
- communicating effectively with, and involving, employees in the development and implementation of the programme;
- creating supportive environments;
- considering incentives to encourage adherence to the programmes, and
- improving self-efficacy of the participants (WHO, 2008b).

Such programmes could help employees to achieve a balance between the demands of their chronic health problem and the demands of their work; and to adapt their self-management skills to changes in organisational and workplace factors. It would also enhance any workplace initiative in managing health and wellbeing by optimising overall quality of working life and by reducing sickness absence, work disability and potential loss of employment.

Conclusion

The studies reviewed in this chapter suggest that self-management behaviours for those with chronic health problems have an important role to play within the workplace and can contribute to improved work productivity, reduced sickness absence and improved wellbeing (for example, Gignac et al, 2002; Hill et al, 2007; Hassan et al, 2009; Munir et al, 2009b, 2009c). This in turn, can enhance a healthy and sustained working life. However, research in this field is still in its infancy and much more evidence, particularly from longitudinal studies, is required to fully examine the potential impact of self-management behaviours at work and workplace self-management intervention programmes. Particularly, research and intervention-based studies are required for those chronic health problems that are not caused by work, but are considered to be work-relevant due to the impact they have on the health, wellbeing and productivity of the workforce (for example, Kessler et al, 2001).

Evidence from healthcare-related self-management programmes has shown that such programmes are effective in improving the health and quality of life of individuals managing a chronic health problem (Barlow et al, 2002). A key strength of these programmes is in empowering such individuals to take responsibility for the management of their health, thereby giving them greater control over their lives (DH, 2001). However, there is a need for further research into the feasibility and effectiveness of workplace self-management programmes and whether these can be successfully integrated into workplaces. Although the workplace intervention studies reviewed here suggest that it is possible to design and implement a self-management programme in the workplace (for example, Varekamp et al, 2008, 2009; Detaille et al, 2010), whether employers can see the benefits of such programmes to their overall business and the feasibility of implementing such initiatives within their organisation is yet to be fully assessed.

This chapter has highlighted some of the key challenges that lie ahead in encouraging employers to integrate self-management programmes into the workplace. Although organisations have an important role to play, it is important for all those involved in managing chronic health problems not to become constrained by self-management programmes but to continue to explore other ways in which policymakers, healthcare, employers and employees themselves can manage chronic health problems.

Further reading

Detaille, S., Heerken, Y.F., Engels, J., van der Gulden, J.W.J. and van Dijk, F.J.H. (2009) 'Common prognostic factors of work disability among employees with a chronic somatic disease: a systematic review of cohort studies', *Scandinavian Journal of Work, Environment and Health*, vol 35, no 4, pp 261-81.

Hill, D., Lucy, D., Tyers, C. and James, L. (2007) *What works at work? Review of evidence assessing the effectiveness of workplace interventions to prevent and manage common health problems*, published for cross-government Health, Work and Wellbeing Unit, London: The Stationery Office.

Lunt, J., Fox, D., Bowen, J., Higgins, G., Crozier, S. and Carter, L. (2007) *Applying the biopsychosocial approach to managing risks of contemporary occupational health conditions: Scoping review*, Health and Safety Laboratory Report, Buxton: Health and Safety Laboratory.

Munir, F., Yarker, J., Randall, R. and Nielsen, K. (2009) 'The influence of employer support on employee management of chronic health conditions at work', *Journal of Occupational Rehabilitation*, vol 19, no 4, pp 333-44.

Varekamp, I., dr Vries, G., Heutink, A. and van Dijk, F. (2008) 'Empowering employees with chronic diseases: development of an intervention aimed at job retention and design of a randomised controlled trial', *BMC Health Services Research*, vol 8, pp 224-32.

References

Allaire, S., Anderson, J. and Meenan, R. (1996) 'Reducing work disability associated with rheumatoid arthritis: identification of additional risk factors and persons likely to benefit from intervention', *Arthritis Care Research*, vol 9, no 5, pp 349-57.

Abraham, C. and Graham-Rowe, E. (2009) 'Are worksite interventions effective in increasing physical activity? A systematic review and meta-analysis', *Health Psychology Review*, vol 3, no 1, pp 108-44.

Baanders, A.N., Andries, F., Rijken, P.M. and Dekker, J. (2001) 'Work adjustments among the chronically ill', *International Journal of Rehabilitation Research*, vol 24, no 1, pp 7-14.

Bandura, A. (1977) 'Toward a unifying theory of behavioral change', *Psychology Review*, vol 84, no 2, pp 191-215.

Bandura, A. (1997) *Self-efficacy: The exercise of control*, New York, NY: Freeman.

Barnes, M.C., Buck, R., Williams, G., Webb, K.L. and Aylward, M. (2008) 'Beliefs about common health problems and work: a qualitative study', *Social Science and Medicine*, vol 67, no 4, pp 657-65.

Barlow, J. (2001) 'How to use education as an intervention in osteoarthritis', in M. Doherty and M. Dougados (eds) *Osteoarthritis. Balliere's best practice research clinical rheumatology*, London: Harcourt Publishers, vol 15, no 4, pp 545-58.

Barlow, J.H., Turner, A.P. and Wright, C.C. (2000) 'A randomised controlled study of the Arthritis Self-Management Programme in the UK', *Education Research Theory and Practice*, vol 15, no 6, pp 665-80.

Barlow, J., Wright, C., Sheasby, J., Turner, A. and Hainsworth, J. (2002) 'Self-management approaches for people with chronic conditions: a review', *Patient Education and Counseling*, vol 48, no 2, pp 177-87.

Bartholomew, L., Parcel, G., Kok, G. and Gottlieb, N. (2006) *Planning health promotion programs: an intervention mapping approach*, San Francisco, CA: Jossey-Bass.

Bhattacharya, J., Choudry, K. and Lakdawalla, D. (2008) 'Chronic disease and severe disability among working-populations', *Medical Care*, vol 46, no 1, pp 92-100.

Black, C. (2008) *Working for a healthier tomorrow*, London: The Stationery Office.

Blokstra, A., Baan, C.A., Boshuizen, H.C., Feenstra, T.L., Hoogeveen, R.T. and Picavet, H.S. (2007) *Impact f the ageing population on burden of disease: Projections of chronic disease prevalence for 2005-2025*. RIVM report 260401004, Bilthoven: National Institute for Public Health and Environment.

Böckerman, P. and Laukkanen, E. (2009) 'What makes you work while you are sick? Evidence from a survey of workers', *European Journal of Public Health*, vol 20, no 1, pp 43-6.

Burton, W.N., Conti, D.J., Chen, C.-Y., Schultz, A.B. and Edington, D.W. (1999) 'The role of health risk factors and disease on worker productivity', *Journal of Occupational Environmental Medicine*, vol 41, no 10, pp 863-77.

Burton, W.N., Pransky, G., Conti, D.J., Chen, C.-Y. and Edington, D.W. (2004) 'The association of medical condition and presenteeism', *Journal of Occupational Environmental Medicine*, vol 46, no 6, pp S38-S45.

Center for the Advancement of Health (2002) *Essential elements of self-management interventions*, Washington DC: Center for the Advancement of Health.

CIPD (Chartered Institute of Personnel Development) (2009) *Absence management: Annual survey report 2009*. London CIPD.

Clark, N.M., Becker, M.H., Janz, N.K., Lorig, K., Rakowski, W. and Anderson, L. (1991) 'Self-management of chronic disease by older adults', *Journal of Aging and Health*, vol 3, no 1, pp 3–27.

Corbin, J. and Strauss, A. (1988) *Unending work and care: Managing chronic illness at home*, San Fransisco, CA: Jossey-Bass.

Currie, S.R. and Wang, J.L. (2004) 'Chronic back pain and major depression in the general Canadian Population', *Pain*, vol 107, no 1-2, pp 54-60.

Curtis, J. (2003) 'Employment and disability in the United Kingdom: an outline of legislative and policy changes', *Work*, vol 20, no 1, pp 45-51.

de Lange, A.H., Taris, T.W., Kompier, M.A.J., Houtman, I.L.D. and Bongers, P.M. (2003) 'The very best of the millennium: longitudinal research and the demand-control-(support) model', *Journal of Occupational Health Psychology*, vol 8, no 4, pp 282-305.

DETR (Department of the Environment, Transport and the Regions) (2000) *Revitalising health and safety: Strategy statement*, Wetherby: Department of the Environment, Transport and the Regions.

DeRidder, D., Geenen, R., Kuijer, R. and van Middendorp, H. (2008) 'Psychological adjustment to chronic disease', *Lancet*, vol 372, no 9634, pp 246-55.

Detaille, S.I., Haafkens, J.A. and van Dijk, F.J.H. (2003) 'What employees with rheumatoid arthritis, diabetes mellitus and hearing loss need to cope at work', *Scandinavian Journal of Work, Environment and Health*, vol 29, no 2, pp 134-42.

Detaille, S., Heerken, Y.F., Engels, J., van der Gulden, J.W.J. and van Dijk, F.J.H. (2009) 'Common prognostic factors of work disability among employees with a chronic somatic disease: a systematic review of cohort studies', *Scandinavian Journal of Work, Environment and Health*, vol 35, no 4, pp 261-281.

Detaille, S.I., van der Gulden, J., Engels, J.A., Heerkens, Y.F. and van Dijk, F. (2010) Using intervention mapping (IM) to develop a self-management programme for employees with a chronic disease in the Netherlands', *BMC Public Health*, vol 10, no 1, p 353.

DH (Department of Health) (1999) *Saving lives: Our healthier nation white paper and reducing health inequalities: An action report*, London: DH.

DH (2001) *The expert patient: A new approach to chronic disease management for the 21st century*, London: DH.

DH (2010) *Improving the health and well-being of people with long term conditions*, London: DH.

Dionne, C.E., Bourbonnias, R., Fremont, P., Rossignol, M., Stock, S.R., Nowen, A., Laroque, I. and Demers, E. (2007) 'Determinants of "return to work in good health" among workers with back pain who consult in primary care settings: a 2-year prospective study', *European Spine Journal*, vol 16, no 5, pp 641-55.

Ditewig, J.B., Blok, H., Havers, J. and van Veenendaal, H. (2010) 'Effectiveness of self-management interventions on mortality, hospital readmissions, chronic heart failure hospitalisation rate and quality of life in patients with chronic heart failure: a systematic review', *Patient Education and Counseling*, vol 78, no 3, pp 297-315.

DWP (Department for Work and Pensions) (2008) *Improving health and work: Changing lives*, London: The Stationery Office.

Feste, C. and Anderson, R.M. (1995) 'Empowerment: from philosophy to practice', *Patient Education and Counseling*, vol 26, no 1-3, pp 139-44.

Franche, R.L., Cullen, K., Clarke, J., Irvin, E., Sinclair, S. and Frank, J. (Institute for Work & Health Workplace-Based RTW Intervention Literature Review Research Team) (2005) 'Workplace-based return-to-work interventions: a systematic review of the quantitative literature', *Journal of Occupational Rehabilitation*, vol 15, no 4, pp 607-31.

Frayne, C.A. and Latham, G.P. (1987) 'Application of social learning theory to employee self-management of attendance', *Journal of Applied Psychology*, vol 72, no 3, pp 387-92.

Gallant, P. (2003) 'The influence of social support on chronic illness self-management: a review and directions for research', *Health Education and Behavior*, vol 30, no 2, pp 170-95.

Gatty, C.M., Turner, M., Buitendorp, D.J. and Bateman, H. (2003) 'The effectiveness of back pain and injury prevention programs in the workplace', *Work*, vol 20, no 3, pp 257-66.

Gibson, P.G., Powell, H., Coughlan, J., Wilson, A.J., Abramson, M., Haywood, P., Bauman, A., Hensley, M.J. Walters, E.H. and Roberts J.J.L. (2002) 'Self-management education and regular practitioner review for adults with asthma (Review)', Cochrane Database of Systematic Reviews 2002, Issue 3, Art No: CD001117, John Wiley and Sons. http://www.thecochranelibrary.com

Gignac, M. (2005) 'Arthritis and employment: an examination of behavioural coping efforts to manage workplace activity limitations', *Arthritis Care & Research*, vol 53, no 3, pp 328-36.

Gignac, M.A.M., Badley, E.M., LaCaille, D., Cott, C.C., Adam, P. and Aslam, H.A. (2002) 'Managing arthritis and employment: making arthritis-related work changes as a means of adaptation', *Arthritis & Rheumatism*, vol 51, no 6, pp 909-16.

Gignac, M.A.M. and Cao, X. (2009) 'Should I tell my employer and coworkers I have arthritis? A longitudinal examination of self-disclosure in the workplace', *Arthritis & Rheumatism*, vol 61, no 12, pp 1753-61.

Glasgow, N.J. and Eakin, E.G. (1998) 'Issues in diabetes self-management', in S.A. Shumaker, E.B. Schron, J.K. Ockene and W.L. McBee (eds) *The handbook of health behaviour change*, New York, NY: Springer, pp 435-61.

Glasgow, N.J., Jeon, Y.-H., Kraus, S. and Pearce-Brown, C.L. (2008) 'Chronic disease self-management support: the way forward for Australia', *Medical Journal of Australia*, vol 189, no 10, pp S14-S16.

Goetzel, Z., Roemer, E.C., Liss-Levinson, R.C. and Samoly, D.K. (2008) *Workplace health promotion: Policy recommendations that encourage employers to support health improvement programs for their workers*, Partnership for Prevention, USA, http://hss.state.ak.us/healthcommission/200905/worksite_health.pdf

Griffiths, C., Motlib, J., Azad, A., Ramsay, J., Eldridge, S., Feder, G., Khanam, R., Munni, R. and Garrett, M. (2005) 'Randomised controlled trial of a lay-led self-management programme for Bangladeshi patients with chronic disease', *British Journal of General Practice*, vol 55, no 520, pp 831-7.

Groeneveld, I.F., Proper, K.I., van der Beek, A.J., Hildebrandt, V.H. and van Mechelen, W. (2010) 'Lifestyle-focused interventions at the workplace to reduce the risk of cardiovascular disease – a systematic review', *Scandinavian Journal of Work Environment and Health*, vol 36, no 3, pp 202-15.

Hackman, J.R. (1987) 'The design of work teams', in J.W. Lorsch (ed) *Handbook of organizational behavior*, Englewood Cliffs, NJ: Prentice Hall, pp 315-42.

Hassan, E., Austin, C., Celia, C., Disley, E., Hunt, P., Marjanovic, S., Shehabi, A., Villalba-van-Dijk, L. and van Stolk, C. (2009) *Health and wellbeing at work in the United Kingdom*, London: The Work Foundation.

Hill, D., Lucy, D., Tyers, C. and James, L. (2007) *What works at work? Review of evidence assessing the effectiveness of workplace interventions to prevent and manage common health problems*, published for cross-government Health, Work and Wellbeing Unit, London: The Stationery Office.

HSE (Health and Safety Executive) (2008) *Improving the health, work and well-being of local communities*, Sudbury: HSE Books, www.hse.gov.uk/lau/laa/laaguide.pdf

HSE (2010) *Health and safety statistics 2008/09*, Sudbury: HSE Books, www.hse.gov.uk/statistics/overall/hssh0809.pdf

Kessler, R.C., Greenberg, P.E., Mickelson, K.D. and Wang, P.S. (2001) 'The effects of chronic medical conditions on work loss and work cutback', *Journal of Occupational and Environmental Medicine*, vol 43, no 3, pp 218-25.

Kessler, R.C., Ormel, J., Demier, O. and Stang, P.E. (2003) 'Comorbid mental disorders account for the role impairment of commonly occurring chronic physical disorders: results from the National Comorbidity Survey', *Journal of Occupational Environmental Medicine*, vol 45, no 12, pp 1257-66.

Kopnina, H. and Haafkens, J.A. (2009) 'Chronically ill employee in the context of organizational culture', *Çalişma ve Toplum*, vol 4, pp 131-52.

Kopnina, H. and Haafkens, J.A. (2010) 'Disability management: organizational diversity and Dutch employment policy', *Journal of Occupational Rehabilitation*, vol 20, no 2, pp 247-55.

Kuijer, W., Groothoff, J.W., Brouwer, S., Geertzen, J.H.B. and Dijkstra, P.U. (2006) 'Prediction of sickness absence in patients with chronic low back pain: a systematic review', *Journal of Occupational Rehabilitation*, vol 16, no 3, pp 439-67.

Kuoppala, J., Lamminpää, A. and Husman, P. (2008) 'Work health promotion, job well-being, and sickness absences – a systematic review and meta-analysis', *Journal of Occupational and Environmental Medicine*, vol 50, no 11, pp 1216-27.

Layard, R. (2005) 'Mental health: Britain's biggest social problem', Paper presented at the No.10 Strategy Unit Seminar on Mental Health, 20 January, www.cabinetoffice.gov.uk/media/cabinetoffice/strategy/assets/mh_layard.pdf

Linton, S. and Halldén, K. (1998) 'Can we screen for problematic back pain? A screening questionnaire for predicting outcome in acute and sub-acute back pain', *The Clinical Journal of Pain*, vol 14, no 3, pp 209-15.

Lerner, D., Amick, B.C., Malspeis, S. and Rogers, W.H. (2000) 'A national survey of health-related work limitations among employed persons in the United States', *Disability and Rehabilitation*, vol 22, no 5, pp 225-32.

Lorig, K.R. and Holman, H.R. (2003) 'Self-management education: history, definition, outcomes, and mechanisms', *Annals of Behavioral Medicine*, vol 26, no 1, pp 1-7.

Lorig, K.R. and Laurin, J. (1985) 'Some notions about the assumptions underlying health education', *Health Education Quarterly*, vol 12, no 3, pp 231-43.

Lorig, K.R., Ritter, P.L., Stewart, A.L., Sobel, D.S., William, B.B., Bandura, A., Gonzalez, V.M., Laurent, D.D. and Holman, H.R. (2001) 'Chronic disease self-management program: 2-year health status and health care utilization outcomes', *Medical Care*, vol 39, no 11, pp 1217-23.

Lunt, J., Fox, D., Bowen, J., Higgins, G., Crozier, S. and Carter, L. (2007) *Applying the biopsychosocial approach to managing risks of contemporary occupational health conditions: Scoping review*, HSL/2007/24, Buxton: Health and Safety Laboratory.

Maher, C.G. (2000) 'A systematic review of workplace interventions to prevent low back pain', *Australian Journal of Physiotherapy*, vol 36, pp 259-69.

Main, C.J., Sullivan, M.J. and Watson, P.J. (2007) 'Pain and work: organisational perspectives', in *Pain management: Practical application of the bio psychosocial perspective in clinical and occupational settings*, Philadelphia, PA: Chuchill Livingstone Elsevier, pp 369-91.

Mancuso, C.L., Paget, S.T. and Charlson, M.E. (2000) 'Adaptations made by rheumatoid arthritis patients to continue working: a pilot study of workplace challenges and successful adaptations', *Arthritis Care and Research*, vol 13, no 2, pp 89-99.

Manz, C.C. and Sims, H.P. (1987) 'Leading workers to lead themselves: the external leadership of self- managing work teams', *Administrative Science Quarterly*, vol 32, no 1, pp 106-29.

Martin, A., Sanderson, K. and Cocker, F. (2009) 'Meta-analysis of the effects of health promotion intervention in the workplace on depression and anxiety symptoms', *Scandinavian Journal of Work Environment and Health*, vol 35, no 1, pp 7-18.

Meijer, E., Sluiter, J., Heyma, A., Sadiraj, K. and Frings-Dresen, M. (2006) 'Cost-effectiveness of multidisciplinary treatment in sick-listed patients with upper extremity musculoskeletal disorders: a randomised, controlled trial with one-year follow-up', *International Archives of Occupational and Environmental Health*, vol 79, no 8, pp 654-64

Michie, S., and Abraham, C. (2004) *Health psychology in practice*, Oxford: British Psychological Society and Blackwell.

Michie, S. and Williams, S. (2003) 'Reducing work related psychological ill health and sickness absence: a systematic literature review', *Occupational Environmental Medicine*, vol 60, no 1, pp 3-9.

Moore, J.E., Von Korff, M., Cherkin, D., Saunders, K. and Lorig, K. (2000) 'A randomized trial of a cognitive-behavioral program for enhancing back pain self care in a primary care setting', *Pain*, vol 88, pp 145-53.

Munir, F., Jones, D., Leka, S. and Griffiths, A. (2005a) 'Work limitations and employer adjustments for employees with chronic illness', *International Journal of Rehabilitation Research*, vol 28, no 2, pp 111-17.

Munir, F., Haslam, C., Long, H., Griffiths, A., Cox, S. and Leka, S. (2005b) 'Managing chronic illness at work: exploring effective strategies for employees and organisations', Report produced for the European Social Fund, Nottingham: University of Nottingham.

Munir, F., Leka, S. and Griffiths, A. (2005c) 'Self-management of chronic illness at work: factors associated with self-disclosure', *Social Science & Medicine*, vol 60, no 6, pp 1397-407.

Munir, F., Yarker, J. and Haslam, C. (2008) 'Sickness absence management: encouraging attendance or risk-taking presenteeism in employees with chronic illness?', *Disability and Rehabilitation*, vol 30, no 19, pp 1461-72.

Munir, F., Yarker, J. and McDermott, H. (2009a) 'Correlates of work ability for those working during or following cancer treatment: a review', *Occupational Medicine*, vol 59, no 6, pp 381-9.

Munir, F., Khan, H., Yarker, J., Haslam, C., Bains, M. and Kalawsky, K. (2009b) 'Self-management of health-behaviors among older and younger workers with chronic illness', *Patient Education & Counselling*, vol 77, no 1, pp 109-15.

Munir, F., Yarker, J., Randall, R. and Nielsen, K. (2009c) 'The influence of employer support on employee management of chronic health conditions at work', *Journal of Occupational Rehabilitation*, vol 19, no 4, pp 333-44.

Munir, F., Nielsen, K. and Carneiro, I.G. (2010) 'Transformational leadership and depressive symptoms', *Journal of Affective Disorders*, vol 120, no1-3, pp 235-9.

Munnell, A. and Libby, J. (2007) *Will people be healthy enough to work longer? Vol 3*, Boston, MA: Center for Retirement Research, pp 1-11.

Newman, S., Steed, L. and Mulligan, K. (2004) 'Self-management interventions for chronic illness', *Lancet*, vol 364, no 9444, pp 1523-36.

Nieuwenhuijsen, K., Verbeek, J., Siemerink, J.C. and Tummers-Nijsen, D. (2003) 'Quality of rehabilitation among workers with adjustment disorders according to practice guidelines; a retrospective cohort study', *Occupational Environmental Medicine*, vol 60, supplement no 1, pp S121-S125.

Plack, K., Herpertz, S. and Petrak, F. (2010) 'Behavioural medicine interventions in diabetes', *Current Opinion in Psychiatry*, vol 23, no 2, pp 131-8.

Reeves, D., Kennedy, A., Fullwood, C., Bower, P., Gardner, C., Gately, C. and Lee, V. (2008) 'Predicting who will benefit from an Expert Patients Programme self-management course', *British Journal of General Practice*, vol 58, no 548, pp 198-203.

Rivilis, I., Van Eerd, D., Cullen, K., Cole, D.C., Irvin, E., Tyson, J. and Mahmood, Q. (2008) 'Effectiveness of participatory ergonomic interventions on health outcomes: a systematic review', *Applied Ergonomics*, vol 39, no 3, pp 342-58.

Roelen, C.A.M., Schreuder, K.J., Koopmans, P.C. and Groothoff, J.W. (2008) 'Perceived job demands relate to self-reported health complaints', *Occupational Medicine*, vol 58, pp 58-63.

Rogers, A. (2009) 'Advancing the expert patient?', *Primary Health Care Research & Development*, vol 10, no1, pp 167-76.

Rogers, A., Kennedy, A., Bower, P., Gardner, C., Gately, C., Lee, V., Reeves, D. and Richardson, G. (2008) 'The United Kingdom Expert Patients Programme: results and implications from a national evaluation', *The Medical Journal of Australia*, vol 189, no 10, pp S21-S24.

Roskes, K., Donders, N.C.G.M. and van der Gulden, J.W.J. (2005) 'Health-related and work-related aspects associated with sick leave: a comparison of chronically ill and non-chronically ill workers', *International Archives of Occupational Environmental Health*, vol 78, no 4, pp 270-8.

Seymour, L. and Grove, B. (2005) *Workplace interventions for people with common mental health problems: Evidence review and recommendations*, London: British Occupational Health Research Foundation.

Stetz, T.A., Stetz, M.C. and Bliese, P.D. (2006) 'The importance of self-efficacy in the moderating effects of social support on stressor-strain relationships', *Work Stress*, vol 20, no 1, pp 49-59.

Taskila, T. and Lindbohm, M.L. (2007) 'Factors affecting cancer survivors' employment and work ability', *Acta Oncologica*, vol 46, no 4, pp 446-51.

van Mierlo, H., Rutte, C.G., Vermunt, J.K., Kompier, M.A.J. and Doorewaard, J.A. (2007) 'A multi-level mediation model of the relationships between team autonomy, individual task design and psychological well-being', *Journal of Occupational and Organizational Psychology*, vol 80, no 4, pp 647-64.

van Mierlo, H., Rutte, C.G., Kompier, M.A.J. and Doorewaard, J.A. (2005) 'Self-managing teamwork and psychological well-being', *Group and Organizational Management*, vol 30, no 2, pp 211-35.

Varekamp, I. and van Dijk, F.J.H. (2010) 'Workplace problems and solutions for employees with chronic diseases', *Occupational Medicine*, vol 60, no 4, pp 287-93.

Varekamp, I., Verbeek, J. and van Dijk, F. (2006) 'How can we help employees with chronic diseases to stay at work? A review of interventions aimed at job retention and based on an empowerment perspective', *International Archives of Occupational Environmental Health*, vol 80, no 2, pp 87-97.

Varekamp, I., dr Vries, G., Heutink, A. and van Dijk, F. (2008) 'Empowering employees with chronic diseases: development of an intervention aimed at job retention and design of a randomised controlled trial', *BMC Health Services Research*, vol 8, pp 224-32.

Varekamp, I., Heutink, A., Selma, L., Koning, C.E.M., de Vries, G. and van Dijk, F.J.H. (2009) 'Facilitating empowerment in employees with chronic disease: qualitative analysis of the process of change', *Journal of Occupational Rehabilitation*, vol 19, no 4, pp 398-408.

Vickers, M. (1997) 'Life at work with "invisible" chronic illness (ICI): the "unseen", unspoken, unrecognised dilemma of disclosure', *Journal of Workplace Learning,* vol 9, no 7, pp 240–52.

Waddell, G. and Aylward, M. (2005) *The scientific and conceptual basis of incapacity benefits,* London: The Stationery Office.

Waddell, G. and Burton, K. (2001) 'Occupational health guidelines for the management of low back pain at work: Evidence review'. *Occupational Medicine,* vol 51, no 2, pp 124-35.

Waddell, G. and Burton, K. (2004) *Concepts of rehabilitation for the management of common health problems,* London: The Stationary Office.

Waddell, G. and Burton, K. (2006) *Is work good for your health and well-being?,* London: The Stationary Office.

Weijman, I., Ros, W.J.G., Rutten, G., Schaufeli, W., Schabracq, M. and Winnubst, J. (2005) 'The role of work-related and personal factors in diabetes self-management', *Patient Education and Counseling,* vol 59, no 1, pp 87-96.

Wesson, M. and Gould, M. (2010) 'Can a "return to work" agenda fit within the theory and practice of CBT for depression and anxiety disorders?', *The Cognitive Behaviour Therapist,* vol 3, no 1, pp 27-42.

Whitehead, M., Clayton, S., Holland, P., Drever, F., Barr, B., Gosling, R., Dahl. E., Van Der Wel, K.E., Westin, S., Burström, B., Nylen, L., Lundberg, O., Diderichsen, F., Thielen, K., Ng, E., Uppal, S. and Chen, W.-H. (2009) *Helping chronically ill or disabled people into work: What can we learn from international comparative analyses?,* Final report to the Public Health Research Programme, Department of Health, Published by University of Liverpool, available from www.york.ac.uk/phrc/PHRC%20C2-06_%20RFR.pdf

Whittemore, R. and Dixon, J. (2008) 'Chronic illness: the process of integration', *Journal of Nursing and Healthcare of Chronic Illness,* vol 17, no 7b, pp 177-87.

WHO (World Health Organization) (2008a) *2008-2013 action plan for the global strategy for the prevention and control of noncommunicable diseases,* Geneva: WHO.

WHO (2008b) *Preventing noncommunicable diseases in the workplace through diet and physical activity,* Geneva: WHO.

Wynne-Jones, G., Buck, R., Porteous, C., Cooper, L., Button, L.A., Main, C.J. and Pillips, C.J. (2010) 'What happens to work if you are unwell? Beliefs and attitudes of managers and employers with musculoskeletal pain in a public sector setting', *Journal of Occupational Rehabilitation,* vol 21, no 1, 32-42.

TWELVE

Case study: organisational change and employee health and wellbeing in the NHS

Julia Gibbs, Wendy Loretto, Tina Kowalski and Stephen Platt

Background

Against the wider background of debates over the positive and negative effects of work on employee wellbeing, there has been a specific interest in organisational change. It is most often suggested that change has a negative effect on employee wellbeing (Ferrie et al, 1998; Tehrani et al, 2007), with concerns expressed over the nature of changes, how they are managed and the rate of change. In particular, a widely held notion that the contemporary employment experience is one of constant change has given legitimacy to focusing on change in its own right. One sector strongly associated with constant change is that of healthcare services, both in the UK (for example, Bach, 2004) and beyond (for example, Schoolfield and Orduna, 1994). Despite this, and despite a growing evidence base that health service employees experience higher levels of mental distress than other working populations (Tennant, 2001; Loretto et al, 2010), remarkably little attention has been paid to managing health service employees through times of change. Existing studies have tended to use quantitative methods (such as Bourbonnais et al, 2005; Hansson et al, 2008). While useful in establishing the nature and extent of stressors associated with organisational change, such research provides limited insight into the ways in which organisational change may affect employee health and how employees adapt and respond to change.

Situated within a multimethod research project in the UK National Health Service (NHS), this chapter reports findings from a qualitative longitudinal study. It aims to explore the dynamic nature of the relationships between organisational change and staff health over the period of a three-year change programme that encompassed the relocation of a key UK hospital trust and major restructuring of service provision. It draws on the demand-control-support (DCS) model (Karasek, 1979; Karasek and Theorell, 1990) to explore how organisational change affected employees' health and investigates how individuals' health trajectories developed over the course of the study.

Change and health

Theorell (1974) was one of the first to suggest that changed work circumstances, such as new responsibilities, work schedules or working relationships, may influence health. Karasek (1979) and Karasek and Theorell (1990) later developed a model that focused on the interactions between 'demands', 'control' and 'support' at work and their role in determining levels of stress-related illnesses ('job strain'). The DCS model suggests that job strain is brought about when people experience a combination of onerous job demands (such as working fast and hard or psychological demands) and low levels of control (lack of authority to make decisions and of opportunity to apply skills). The model also suggests that social support may facilitate coping patterns and act as a 'buffering' mechanism between psychological stress and adverse health outcomes. This includes both 'socio-emotional' support (social and emotional integration, trust and cohesion between co-workers, supervisors and others) and 'instrumental social support' (extra resources or assistance with tasks given to employees by co-workers or supervisors).

While the DCS model has been widely used and (for the most part) positively evaluated in the health literature, its application to change situations has so far been limited. Nevertheless, some studies have examined the effects of various components in relations to change at work. Thus, in relation to support, Väänänen and colleagues (2004) found organisational and supervisor support to be an important influence on staff health during organisational change. On the other hand, Terry and colleagues (1996) suggested that co-worker support may not be so influential because it cannot provide resources to cope with demands. Furthermore, Begley (1998) suggested that co-workers may be restricted in their capacity to provide support when they are also emotionally upset about organisational change. Bordia and colleagues (2004) highlighted the control dimension of the model, suggesting that the negative impact of organisational change on psychological health arises because of uncertainty, which is related to lack of control.

Another limitation of the application of the model to date is that it has been rather narrow in its construction of demands, controls and supports, generally limiting them to the employment context. However, a substantial body of research (see Loretto et al, 2005) points to the importance of social support outside work – most often from friends and family – in influencing work demands and ways in which to cope with such demands. The interface between organisational change, home life and health have been further explored by Burke and Greenglass (2001), who found that nurses reporting increased workload or threats to job security as a result of work restructuring were also more likely to report higher work–family conflict, which in turn reduced job satisfaction and had a negative effect on their psychological health.

Thus, a key principle of this study was the importance of adopting a holistic approach when examining how organisational change affects employee health and wellbeing. This was to be achieved by considering factors outside, as well as within, the workplace and the interaction between external and internal influences.

Case study of employee health and change

The case study reported here is part of a wider, multimethod prospective study of organisational change within the UK NHS (see Loretto et al, 2010 for results from the quantitative element of the study). A three-year qualitative study of organisational change and staff health was carried out in one UK hospital trust and involved a combination of in-depth interviewing, observation and documentary analysis techniques. The findings presented here will focus on restructuring that took place within the Reproductive Medicine Directorate. As part of the restructuring process, and within the context of the wider NHS emphasis on integrated patient care teams, maternity services (MS) were being redesigned to break down the traditional primary–secondary care divide. Midwives were to be brought together with other health professionals, notably hospital doctors and GPs, and former community midwives and hospital midwives were to be members of integrated teams. The strategy was intended to deliver a patient-focused service; old boundaries between midwives who delivered only antenatal care and those who focused on postnatal care, and between hospital-based and community-based midwives, were to disappear. As a result, teams were extensively reconfigured and roles and the power balance between team members had to be renegotiated. An additional complication was the move of secondary care services from a city-centre location to a new out-of-town hospital site at the same time as the new maternity services strategy was being implemented.

During the first year of the study, preparations were under way for the hospital relocation; by the second year, staff in Reproductive Medicine had moved to the new site. During the period of the study, changes to MS were gradually rolled out team by team. However, before the roll-out was completed, many staff demanded revisions to the strategy, with the support of their trade union. This led to the strategy being put on hold at a point when some teams were operating according to new systems of work while others continued to operate under existing procedures. This situation continued for many months while the strategy was reviewed. Revisions to the strategy had not been completely finalised and implemented by the end of this study. However, steps were being taken that involved further significant changes, including movement of staff between teams.

Interviews were conducted with four teams within MS, incorporating midwives, clinical support workers and administrators at three time points over a two-year period. The interviews were in the form of semi-structured discussions, which encouraged staff to share their own perceptions of change and its influences on their health, with interviewers probing the points they raised. A topic guide was used to prompt discussions on the broad themes of: respondents' changing work roles and responsibilities, including the demands made of them and resources available; problems or challenges encountered and resolutions or coping strategies; sources of social support; the interface between work and home; and perceptions of the relationships between workplace change and individual health experiences (physical, psychosocial and health-relevant behaviours).

The findings are presented in two sections. The first section, based on interviews with all four teams included in the study, aims to provide an overview of the changes experienced by staff and the perceived impact on their health. In the second section, an in-depth analysis of data generated in interviews with nine members of one of the midwifery teams is intended to enhance understanding of longitudinal pathways between organisational change and staff health. Together, these sections seek to provide an integrated approach to studying change (Walker et al, 2007), linking content, process, contextual and individual factors.

Findings

Section 1: overview of health effects of changes

Following Walker and colleagues (2007), we found that individuals reported *content* issues relating to the nature of the changes being implemented, and *process* issues arising from the actions taken by themselves or others to implement the changes. We address each of these in turn, drawing particular attention to how these influenced work demands and control over work. In addition, we explore support, a key part of the internal *context*.

Content of change: influences of altered circumstances at work

The most frequently mentioned circumstances were:

- working hours
- organisation of work
- tasks
- workload intensification
- work environment and work location
- resources.

Working hours

Changes perceived as involving more adverse shift patterns were said to increase tiredness, sleep problems and stress. Some staff who had previously chosen roles that matched their preferences for particular working patterns were upset when these were altered as a result of organisational change. Interviewees also reported that their sense of wellbeing was affected by the ease with which they could combine home and work life commitments. Some found altered working hours disruptive and stressful. Some staff had little advance warning of changes to their shifts and their routines, which they found stressful.

Organisation of work

Staff reported feelings of frustration resulting from the belief that new systems of work would have adverse effects on the service that they could provide. Some said that new work systems affected their perceptions of personal and client safety, as well as their self-confidence and stress levels. For example, shift patterns and allocation determined the frequency with which they could conduct and master particular skills.

Tasks

Additional demands, such as learning new skills or transferring a service to a new site, were sometimes described as stimulating, even though these could also be tiring. When the MS strategy was introduced, some staff initially welcomed opportunities to learn new techniques and update their skills, finding this challenging and rewarding. However, others felt some new requirements were stressful and physically demanding. Furthermore, staff were not motivated to conduct new approaches that they perceived might have adverse consequences for service quality.

Workload intensification

Staff from all the teams reported feeling stressed and tired at work and home when their workload increased as a result of changes to staff:patient ratios, the pace of work, numbers of breaks and overtime. Many also became anxious about the quality of their work when they had to respond to non-stop intensive demands. Prolonged periods of staff shortages were said to have particularly adverse effects on wellbeing. Many staff said the kinds of pressures described below contributed to sickness absence:

> 'Just before I went off sick, I was due annual leave but I can remember feeling very run down and feeling that I just maybe needed a couple of days off, just to build myself up.... I remember looking at the off-duty rota and didn't see anywhere I could get some time off.... And then I think somebody else had gone off sick and I had to take up some of their workload as well.... I was already feeling bombarded without the added strain.... It was like juggling some balls and then somebody throwing me a whole load of other balls and they just all fell down.... I just couldn't go on, it was far too much worry.' (Respondent 47, Time 3)

Work environment and work location

A number of staff said that their general wellbeing was affected by aspects of their physical work environment. Many staff involved in the hospital move were very pleased with their new working environment, but others experienced problems relating to space, light, heating and ventilation. Health was also perceived to be influenced by the locality and accessibility of their workplace, because this affected the length of the working day and tiredness levels.

Resources

Many staff from all the teams reported that resources for patients were generally better at the new hospital than at the old site, but some felt that insufficient attention had been given to features such as appropriate administrative workspaces and rest and catering amenities, which were important for staff wellbeing. Concerns were expressed with regard to the reduction in the number of patient beds. Respondents reported that they frequently had to move women out of the hospital earlier than they would have liked. On occasion, this made their work more stressful, particularly when they had to contend with adverse reactions from patients and their families.

Influence of organisational change processes

It was clear from the interviews that the processes relating to planning, communicating and implementing change were felt to influence health. Prior to relocation, the dominant themes were anxiety about which aspects of their jobs were going to alter and worry about how they would contend with the uncertainties of the changes. Some also felt a loss of control over their work when changes were pending, because they believed that positive aspects of their current service might be stopped or altered as new systems were introduced.

> 'We had a lot of people stressed ... everyone was uptight with the move ... a bit uncertain, nobody knew where they were going.' (Respondent 19, Time 3)

As changes began to be planned and implemented, additional short-term demands were made of staff, such as preparatory meetings and sorting out the logistics of moving premises or new strategic approaches. These placed additional strain on staff:

> 'There were lots of sleepless nights and waking up in the middle of the night in a sweat because it was dreadful ... "What about such and such, oh I haven't thought of that".... You know, I got quite panicky feelings at times.' (Respondent 1, Time 1)

Operating in unfamiliar situations at work was stressful for some staff, as was adapting home life responsibilities around new requirements. People had to apply extra effort as they learnt to carry out new approaches and routines at work and at home. When people felt able to adjust, such changed circumstances became the new norm and anxieties gradually dissipated. However, staff continued to feel stressed when there were particular aspects of their new circumstances that were found to be problematic, such as hours of work or certain working practices. Furthermore, when there was continuing uncertainty about the possibility of further revisions to the strategy, it was difficult to stabilise new working patterns and practices. Many staff reported feeling increasingly stressed and weary when uncertainties persisted for prolonged periods without resolution, as was the case during the attempted implementation of the MS strategy, described in the following extracts.

> 'Oh, it's building up and building up. And the complete uncertainty about everything – where you're going to be, what's happening, what hours we're going to be told to do, all these sort of things have been hanging over us for several years now. And you're told something suddenly ... it all seems to be ... happening in like two or three weeks' time.... But then nothing came of that the last time ... we were told we had to go into the hospital and cover the labour ward ... but then nothing ... that seems to have been put on hold. But it's still hanging over you, because it could be another phone call tomorrow.' (Respondent 45, Time 3)

> 'When people are stressed, they succumb to genuine things ... I think people succumb to colds and it just becomes too much and they're brought down, their resistance is lower ... that, of course, adds an extra stress on the rest of the people who're trying to do the work that is not being done by those that are missing. But I don't think that's new ... but it has been very evident since this strategy.... There's been a rise in sick leave.... People feel the need to take a couple of days off when previously they might have struggled in.' (Respondent 44, Time 3)

A common feeling among staff, when their concerns were unheeded during periods of organisational change, was that they were not valued.

> 'I feel we're all commodities and if you are giving what they want, then you're fine but I don't feel that we're looked at as people any longer.... As soon as the system needs to

change, then they don't mind what happens to the staff.' (Respondent 31, Time 3)

Some staff affected by the MS strategy became actively involved in calling for revisions through collective action, supported by their professional union. They succeeded in halting the full implementation of the strategy and, after a long period of negotiation, achieved some fundamental changes to the strategy. However, this period of resistance was reported as being stressful, as it involved conflict between staff who resisted key elements of the strategic change, and managers who wanted to implement it fully. Conflicts also arose between staff teams that had already begun implementation and those that had not. Some staff who had embraced the new MS strategy reported a loss of control when they realised that they would be the ones most adversely affected by further revisions.

> 'I couldn't get over last year, how massive the change was that we went through ... and I thought we'd got round that fairly well ... and now to be faced with this ... which has all been brought on by other people, is really difficult. I feel really frustrated about it.... It feels like it could really get out of our control now. We're just ... at the whim of other people ... and it's not been imposed by management, it's been imposed by colleagues, in a sense, and I feel very angry with them.' (Respondent 1, Time 2)

Influence of support from work and home situations

Many people valued supportive working relations with colleagues who pulled together to face difficulties arising out of change initiatives. However, this kind of support was said to be limited in its capacity to ease the stress of problematic changes. When change processes involved breaking up established teams, people had to develop new relationships as well as adapting to new working practices. Changes to team structures, work schedules and shifts affected the regularity with which people worked together, and some staff said this influenced the degree of support available to them. Even when staff offered support to one another, they could still feel overwhelmed when they felt they lacked the resources to address the problems at hand. In such situations, staff felt that management support was the key to improving morale as well as addressing practical problems.

'Particularly those several months where it was really bad, we did work well together, helping each other as much as we could. But I'd say we also felt very frustrated because one of our colleagues who eventually went on sick leave with stress, all the signs were very obvious ... there was nothing we could do to help.... Our hands were tied because we were all in the same boat.... We feel very remote from management. I don't think that they really know what our day-to-day workload is like ... our manager never came up to see us here.... I don't feel that we had much support ... a bit of morale boost would've been helpful, maybe a visit to see us up here would've meant something to us at the time, as well as some practical help.' (Respondent 45, Time 1)

During times of change, some staff turned to other work-related support mechanisms outside their line management structures. Several reported that in-house occupational health practitioners had been able to assess their changed work situations and advise and support them on circumstances that posed health risks.

'I've gone through Occupational Health, because I just couldn't see how, if I was redeployed out of there a few years ago as not suitable to be working there, then how could they put me back in.... Occupational Health and Personnel have been really good.' (Respondent 46, Time 3)

Family and friends outside work were also often involved in responding to the consequences of organisational change. Sometimes they provided practical support, such as taking on childcare responsibilities, to help individuals adjust to changes to shift patterns or journey times to work. Many also offered emotional support to staff who were struggling with new work conditions.

'[The travelling has] cut into my time.... My Mum comes to watch the kids ... I couldn't do it without her ... I would've been forced into getting another job.' (Respondent 34, Time 2)

'You can always talk things over with somebody and ... get things in proportion.' (Respondent 12, Time 3)

However, new work demands could put a strain on relationships when they infringed on personal time and home commitments. Partners' and children's lives were sometimes adversely affected by organisational change requirements, and this was an additional source of stress for many staff.

These accounts provide evidence that both the substance and the process of change affected staff health. As expected, situations associated with increasing demands and partial or full loss of control resulted in poorer reported health outcomes. To some extent, these effects were ameliorated by support received from colleagues and family and friends, but on occasions these potential supports added to the strain placed on individuals. This section in the main confirms existing findings from the quantitative element of this study (and from other studies relying on quantitative methods), but also begins to illustrate ways in which individuals have agency and are not merely passive recipients of change. Moreover, the analysis starts to suggest that effects of organisational change on employee health are not merely one-way. Accounts illustrate the ways in which changes in health shape individuals' subsequent responses to change. To explore these processes in more detail, and to fully exploit the longitudinal nature of the data, we turn to individuals' health trajectories over the period of the study.

Section 2: health trajectories and change

Individual trajectories were constructed by returning to the original interview transcripts for one entire team. These aimed to review how each person's experience of change and the effects of change on their health altered during the course of the study.

Vignettes were subsequently derived for each individual in this sub-sample. Additional information on their mental health status was collected via completion at each interview of the General Health Questionnaire (12-item version (GHQ-12); Goldberg, 1978). The GHQ-12 is a standardised scale for measuring psychological ill health and screening tool for assessing the likelihood of psychiatric illness. Scale scores range from 0-12, and a score of 4+ is taken to signify a high likelihood of suffering from a psychiatric illness ('caseness'). The results are provided in Table 12.1 below.

This pattern of GHQ scores suggested four different mental health trajectories:

- trajectory 1: health improvement over the time of the study;
- trajectory 2: temporary health improvement and subsequent decline;

Table 12.1: Interviewees' GHQ scores

Respondent number	Full time (FT) or part time (PT)	Original (O) or new (N) team member	GHQ scores (* = GHQ case)		
			Year 1	Year 2	Year 3
1	FT	O	0	0	6*
2	FT	O	9*	11*	0
3	PT	N	0	1	8*
6	FT	O	12*	0	12*
8	FT	O	7*	0	6*
16	PT	N	0	0	0
24	FT	O	7*	6*	1
31	FT	O	0	0	3
35	FT	N	0	0	No interview
37	PT	N	0	4*	8*

- trajectory 3: health decline over the time of the study;
- trajectory 4: good health throughout the study.

The following findings present an exploration of the trajectories of each of these groups using the vignettes. Before presenting these in some detail, we consider the context of the changes experienced by team members.

Team background and context

Before organisational changes were introduced, the team had focused on community midwifery, with only occasional visits to the labour ward to update skills or to accompany patients. Team members conducted most of their work on the basis of a five-day week, generally during normal working hours (starting after 8am and finishing before 6pm), with some exceptions, such as evening sessions with patients. They also had on-call duties that were covered through a rota system.

The team was among the initial set of community teams to implement new strategic changes. The organisational change situation involved new shift patterns, with each team member conducting community midwifery duties on their short seven- to eight-hour shifts and labour ward duties on their long 12.5-hour shifts. The new labour ward responsibilities meant that staff had to do night shifts on a regular basis, working more nights than under the previous on-call system. Furthermore, days and hours of shifts varied from week to week for many staff, which was a big change from the regular working hours under the old system.

As part of the strategic changes, the team was expanded: some of the interviewees were long-standing team members, while others had only recently joined. Thus, they were undergoing different change experiences, according to the contrasts between their previous and current work situations.

Shortly after the implementation had begun, other teams and some staff in this team met with their union because they were very unhappy about the changes. There was a long series of meetings between staff, union representatives and managers and the strategy was reviewed. Over the three-year study, there continued to be uncertainty about how the changes already implemented in this team would be revised and which team members would be redeployed to other teams as a result of the revisions.

Trajectory 1: improved mental health (respondents 2 and 24)

Both participants in this group were long-standing team members. They looked back fondly to the time when they were part of a much smaller, close-knit and supportive team and believed that patients were receiving a worse service as a result of the changes. They were stressed by the increased demands from the new shift system, which they found tiring and highly disruptive to their home lives. They resented being forced to return to this unsociable shift system that they thought they had left behind earlier in their careers. Their families were very upset by the changing shift patterns and the participants found it difficult to juggle them with their childcare responsibilities. Loss of control was also articulated through financial pressures – it cost more to travel to the new hospital location. Both respondents also had to give up regular activities, including exercise classes, which had a negative impact on physical health. They were also contending with stressors that were not work-related.

By year two, both respondents had been signed off work, one for some weeks, the other for some months. Supportive managers, in turn supported by the occupational health team, GPs and the union, were the key to breaking this downward trajectory. Through these routes, both respondents were able to move to other teams that had not gone through the same changes. This reintroduced control and reduced demands (both in-work demands and those affecting work–life balance, especially shift work and travel-to-work time and expense). However, one respondent made it very clear she would consider a change of career should her new team be forced to implement the changes.

Trajectory 2: temporary improvement in mental health, followed by subsequent decline (respondents 6 and 8)

Again, both members of this group were long-standing team members: one was a midwife and the other was an administrator. While the midwife emphasised the changing shift system as being particularly disruptive and stressful, the administrator was not affected directly by this change. However, she found the declining morale of her team colleagues led to them providing less support to her which in turn resulted in sleep problems, thereby having a negative effect on her health. The midwife also reported problems with sleeping. Prior to the second interview, both had been signed off work and had received support during that time – from colleagues, from the occupational health team and from GPs – which enabled them to take control over some aspects of their changing work lives. The midwife returned to more regular and shorter shifts, while the administrator negotiated some flexibility over her hours. This helped both respondents to manage their work and family commitments. However, these improvements were short-lived. By year three, both respondents reported that the continuing changes had led to a very negative and damaging atmosphere within the team. The original team was fragmented (mentioned earlier) and there was a rapid decline in support from colleagues.

Trajectory 3: decline in mental health (respondents 1, 3 and 37)

One respondent was a long-standing member of the team, while the others were recent recruits. All reported feeling rather positive towards the changes at the outset. The key to this was that they felt they had some control over their patterns of working. In particular, the newer recruits who had come from a hospital setting were used to working the longer shifts and so this did not represent a significant change to them. The long-standing team member had also been actively engaged with the implementation of the changes. However, by year two, all were finding the shifts tiring and reported difficulties with fitting in shifts with their home lives. Despite these difficulties, all mentioned a high degree of support, both from outside work (families and friends) and from colleagues. The long-standing team member also continued to be involved with the change processes by developing relationships with the other teams to try to solve problems emerging from the changes. However, by year three, her feelings of control had diminished and she felt she had no support from management or the other team members. She felt she was 'clinging on', with support from friends and family. By year three, the demands of the new ways of working had exhausted the newer team members, and this was severely affecting their health and the quality of their life outside work. They were both considering giving up their jobs.

Trajectory 4: good mental health (respondents 16, 31 and 35)

This group also comprised two new recruits to the team (one of whom worked part time) and one long-standing member. As with the previous group, the new recruits had previously worked long shifts in the hospital setting and so the new shifts did not represent a significant change for them. The long-standing team member was more positive than some of her colleagues. Her children were older and so she felt that the shifts did not have as negative an impact on her home life as they might have done. However, again by year two, all reported dissatisfaction with the demands the shifts were placing on them. All were tired and they felt that their control of the situation was diminished because staffing levels were so low, with other colleagues signed off sick. Despite problems with instrumental support, all commented on the high levels of emotional support from colleagues, but it was the high level of support received from families that enabled them to be relatively positive. They also reported introducing control into their situations, albeit in different ways. The long-standing team member was able to renegotiate her shifts so that she had an extra day off each week and she had also moved closer to work to reduce commuting time, while the part-time midwife attributed her coping to not being as badly affected by the changes as full-time colleagues. She did, however, express concerns about lack of control in that she now had to drive home alone after nightshifts. The third member of this group exerted control by moving teams – she reported that her new team was much more supportive and cohesive (she was not interviewed in year three). By year three, the two who had not moved were anxious about their futures. Both felt angry with management for the continued changes and lack of consultation and did not feel valued. They both reported feeling cynical and the long-term member was having problems sleeping as a result.

Discussion and conclusion

From these trajectories, it is quite clear that, despite individual differences, changes in demands, control and support and the interactions between them had profound effects on the health of staff experiencing organisational change. In line with Karasek and Theorell's

(1990) DCS model, the analysis of these accounts demonstrates that individuals faced with rising demands, loss of control and reduced support were the most likely to report health problems both in the interviews and as indicated by their score on the GHQ. However, our findings go beyond the DCS model in several ways. First, all the respondent accounts demonstrate the importance of life outside work in influencing demands, control and support. The main emphasis in the work–life balance literature has been on the way that life outside of work makes demands on work, whereas our findings illustrate the very important ways in which an employee's family and friends may enable them to exert control over their work situation, including coping with organisational change.

Second, the longitudinal nature of our data also facilitates some insight into applying the DCS model over time. We highlight how the elements and relationships between them are not static. For example, the support received from colleagues at the outset was often eroded as the organisational change proceeded. The exertion of control in itself could turn into a demand over time and thus have a negative impact on health.

In terms of adding to understanding the processes of organisational change, a third key finding was that individuals were able to exert ultimate control by removing themselves from the situation. This had a direct effect on their mental health. As we argued at the beginning of this chapter, the role of the individual in change outcomes has been neglected. One of the few models in the change management literature to consider individuals is the Kubler-Ross (1978) model, which was originally developed to describe adaptation and response to bereavement. Schoolfield and Orduna (1994) have utilised this framework in analysing nurses' responses to change in the US, showing how nurses went through the classic stages of denial, anger, bargaining, chaos, resignation, readiness and re-emergence. They also mapped this on to Lewins' (1947) classic 'unfreeze, change, refreeze' model. While such an emphasis on individuals is welcome, our research indicates that it needs to be rethought and extended. First, it implies that the individual employee is passive in their receipt of change and reaction to it. As we have shown, this is far from the case. Many of our respondents were active agents in shaping change and the ways in which changes influenced aspects of their working and non-working lives, including their health. Second, there is a further implicit assumption that all change is positive and that once people can see the benefits they will adapt and re-energise, thus leading to 'successful' change. Successful adaptation for the individual thus becomes synonymous with adopting the change. However, when we examine the health outcomes, it may well be that success for the individual, that is, preserving or improving their health or maintaining standards of service, means avoiding the change (such as moving teams) or actively trying to disrupt the change (intervening in the strategy).

Considering our findings as a whole leads us to conceptualise the effects of change on individual employees in a more holistic and interactive manner than has hitherto been done. Based on our research findings, Figure 12.1 summarises these processes and relationships.

Staff health is not usually the first issue to be considered when new organisational changes are being developed in health services. There are many other strategic issues, such as improving patient care or enhancing efficiency, that compete for attention. However, it can be seen from these real-life examples that staff health may be affected in many different ways by organisational change. Staff health may also have important consequences for the service outcomes of strategic changes. We therefore feel that staff health is an essential factor for managers to take into consideration when they are planning and implementing organisational change. If staff health issues are neglected, strategic plans may run into difficulties as a result of increasing staff sickness absence and higher staff turnover.

Figure 12.1: Relationships between organisational change and health

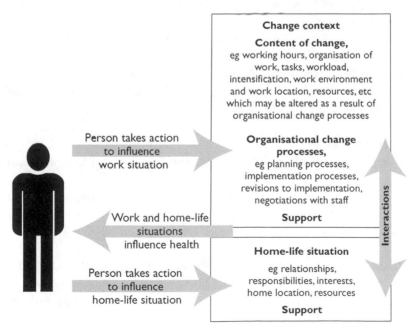

Obviously, this research was carried out in one particular context within the health services and would benefit from further investigation in different organisational settings. However, many of the key processes identified in the literature on organisational change and health were found to be at work within this study context. We believe that our conceptualisation of the longitudinal interactions between individuals and their work and home-life processes during times of organisational change may have wider resonance in a variety of sectors undergoing comparable levels of structural change. If, as was noted at the beginning of this chapter, change is constant and reflects the reality of contemporary employment, managing change successfully is crucial for employee *and* organisational wellbeing.

Further reading

Bach, S. (2004) *Employment relations and the health service:The management of reforms*, London: Routledge.

Boorman, S. (2009) *NHS health and well-being, final report*, Leeds: Department of Health. Available from: www.nhshealthandwellbeing. org/FinalReport.html.

Loretto, W., Popham, F., Platt, S., Pavis, S., Hardy, G., Macleod, L. and Gibbs, J. (2005) 'Assessing psychological wellbeing: a holistic investigation of NHS employees', *International Review of Psychiatry*, vol 17, no 5, pp 329–36.

Loretto, W., Platt, S. and Popham, F. (2010) 'Workplace change and employee mental
health: results from a longitudinal study', *British Journal of Management*, vol 21, no 2, pp 526–40.

Tehrani, N., Humpage, S., Willmott, B. and Haslam, I. (2007) *What's happening with wellbeing at work?*, London: Chartered Institute of Personnel and Development.

References

Bach, S. (2004) *Employment relations and the health service:The management of reforms*, London: Routledge.

Begley, T.M. (1998) 'Coping strategies as predictors of employee distress and turnover after an organisational consolidation: a longitudinal study', *Journal of Occupational and Organizational Psychology*, vol 71, no 4, pp 305–29.

Bordia, P., Hobman, E., Jones, E., Gallois, C. and Callan, V. (2004) 'Uncertainty during organisational change: types, consequences and management strategies', *Journal of Business and Psychology*, vol 18, no 4, pp 507–532.

Bourbonnais, R., Brisson, C., Vezina, M., Masse, B. and Blanchette, C. (2005) 'Psychosocial work environment and certified sick leave among nurses during organizational change and downsizing', *Relations Industrielles (IndustrialRelations)*, vol 60, no 3, pp 483-509.

Burke, R. and Greenglass, E. (2001) 'Hospital restructuring stressors, work-family concerns and psychological well-being among nursing staff', *Community, Work & Family*, vol 4, no 1, pp 49-62.

Ferrie, J., Shipley, M., Marmot, M., Stansfeld, S. and Smith, G. (1998). 'The health effects of major organisational change and job insecurity', *Social Science and Medicine*, vol 46, no 2, pp 243-54.

Goldberg, D. (1978) *General Health Questionnaire (12-item)*, Windsor: NFER-Nelson.

Hansson, A., Vingard, E., Arnetz, B. and Anderzen, I. (2008) 'Organizational change, health and sick leave among health care employees: a longitudinal study measuring stress markers, individual and work site factors', *Work and Stress*, vol 22, no 1, pp 69-80.

Karasek, R.A. (1979) 'Job demands, job decision latitude, and mental strain: implications for job redesign', *Administrative Science Quarterly*, vol 24, no 2, pp 285-307.

Karasek, R. and Theorell, T. (1990) *Healthy work: Stress, productivity, and the reconstruction of working life*, New York, NY: Basic Books.

Kubler-Ross, E. (1978) *To live until we say goodbye*, Englewood Cliffs, NJ: Prentice-Hall.

Lewins, K. (1947) 'Frontiers in group dynamics: concept, method and reality', *Human Relations*, vol 1, no 1, pp 5-42.

Loretto, W., Popham, F., Platt, S., Pavis, S., Hardy, G., Macleod, L. and Gibbs, J. (2005) 'Assessing psychological wellbeing: a holistic investigation of NHS employees', *International Review of Psychiatry*, vol 17, no 5, pp 329-36.

Loretto, W., Platt, S. and Popham, F. (2010) 'Workplace change and employee mental health: results from a longitudinal study' *British Journal of Management*, vol 21, no 2, pp 526-40.

Tehrani, N., Humpage, S., Willmott, B. and Haslam, I. (2007) *What's happening with wellbeing at work?*, London: Chartered Institute of Personnel and Development.

Tennant, C. (2001) 'Work-related stress and depressive disorders', *Journal of Psychosomatic Research*, vol 51, no 5, pp 697-704.

Schoolfield, M. and Orduna., A. (1994) 'Understanding staff nurse responses to change: utilization of a grief-change framework to facilitate intervention', *Clinical Nurse Specialist*, vol 8, no 1, pp 57-62.

Terry, D.J., Callan, V.J. and Sartori, G. (1996) 'Employee adjustment to an organizational merger: stress, coping and intergroup differences', *Stress Medicine*, vol 12, no 2, pp 105-22.

Theorell, T. (1974) 'Life events before and after the onset of a premature myocardial infarction', in B.S. Dohrenwend and B.P. Dohrenwend (eds) *Stressful life events: Their nature and effects*, New York, NY: John Wiley & Sons.

Väänänen, A., Pahkin, K., Kalimo, R. and Buunk, B. (2004) 'Maintenance of subjective health during a merger: the role of experienced change and pre-merger social support at work in white and blue collar workers', *Social Science and Medicine*, vol 58, no 10, pp 1903-15.

Walker, H.J., Armenakis, A.A. and Bernerth, J.B. (2007) 'Factors influencing organizational change efforts: an integrative investigation of change content, context, process and individual differences', *Journal of Organizational Change Management*, vol 20, no 6, pp 761-73.

THIRTEEN

Education and training in the workplace

Chris Phillipson

Introduction

Addressing new challenges for training and education in the workplace has become a significant area of attention. Extending working life is now a major theme of public policy across Western Europe and the United States (Vickerstaff, 2010). The over-50s are being targeted as 'the new work generation' (OECD, 2006; EHRC, 2010) in response to demographic and economic pressures – labour force projections indicating that by 2021 around 32% of the working-age population will be aged 50 and over. The forces driving this attention to older workers are relatively easy to sketch; more complex will be developing satisfactory responses to supporting training and learning across the different types of employment emerging in post-industrial economies.

This focus on older workers is the result of a number of recent measures aimed at addressing the challenges posed by societies with ageing populations. First, and almost certainly foremost, is the expected raising of state pension age (SPA) to 66 for men and women by 2020, this posing the challenge of improving the supply of suitable jobs while ensuring effective career development for all grades of workers (TAEN, 2011). Second, is the phasing out of the Default Retirement Age, which will remove the right of employers to retire people on grounds of reaching a particular age (currently 65). Third, is the move from defined benefit (DB) to defined contribution (DC) pensions, which has put pressure on some older workers to delayed retirement (Phillipson, 2009). In addition, the desirability of early retirement is being increasingly challenged, with the social and personal costs of leaving work ahead of SPA emphasised in documents such as *Winning the generation game* (PIU, 2000) and *Opportunity age* (DWP, 2005).

The policy of extending working lives has been a significant outcome of the debate concerning the economic sustainability of ageing populations, and reflects in large measure these concerns. In essence, the discussion has shifted from focusing on *early retirement/early exit* to identifying *pathways into work or maintaining older people in employment*, with particular encouragement given to work beyond SPA. The aim is to reverse the trend – characteristic of the 1980s and 1990s – whereby large numbers of older workers left work ahead of SPA, and where early retirement came to be accepted as a normal event in the life-course (Marshall et al, 2001).

The extent of the decline in employment among older workers – especially over the period from the 1970s through to the early 1990s – is important to recognise, especially given ambitions to removing barriers to employment. The dominant pattern over this period was the declining age of exit from the labour force – a trend that accelerated during the 1970s and 1980s (Laczko and Phillipson, 1991). Even up to 1971, 93% of men in Britain aged 55-59 and 83% aged 60-64 were economically active, with around 19% of men working on after SPA. By 1989, however, the rate for men aged 55-59 had dropped to 79.8% and for those 60-64 to 54.6% (Phillipson, 1993). Put another way, while in 1950 the average age of exit (for men) from employment was 67.2 years, with 18 years spent in retirement, by 1990 average age had dropped to 63.5% with 27 years now spent in the period following cessation of work (Pensions Commission, 2004).

Over the course of the 1990s, with the move out of economic recession, the pattern of early exit from work went into reverse with increases in economic activity for men and women in their 50s and 60s. Despite, however, the upward move in employment rates, most people once reaching SPA (nearly 90% according to the UK Labour Force Survey (LFS)) become classified as 'economically inactive', and this still applies to around one in four of those aged 50-plus (with ill health or sickness an important component). Moreover, all those in the 50-plus age group are affected by the evolution of the more complex transitions associated with what Giddens (1991) has defined as a post-industrial life course. Here, the evidence suggests that the apparent stability of work-retirement transitions in the 1950s and 1960s (limited in any event to men in secure occupations) was almost certainly a brief interlude in what has always been an unsettled period of the life-course. The emergence in these decades of a 'crisp' transition from employment to retirement at a standard age (for example, 60 or 65) has been undercut by transformations in economic and social policy. Increasingly, departure from work is 'blurred' rather than 'crisp' and may involve a number of moves in and out of paid work (Phillipson, 2002).

Given the above context, this chapter examines the implications for education and training of policies to extend working life. Developing robust support for workers in these areas will, arguably, have a significant impact on health and wellbeing in the workplace. Against this, the evidence to date suggests continuing problems for many groups of workers in accessing good-quality training over the life-course (Phillipson and Smith, 2005).

This chapter examines three main areas:

- the sociological and economic context for understanding changes affecting older workers and retirement;
- research on trends relating to education and training in the workplace; and
- policy initiatives for improving access to training within and beyond employment.

Training and older workers: theoretical frameworks

Training and education would, at first sight, appear to be priority areas, given the focus on retaining older workers in employment, alongside the need to promote health and wellbeing. In reality, however, this area has suffered considerable neglect over the years – despite moves in public policy emphasising the value of older employees. Understanding the reasons behind this marginalisation has been complicated by the limited use of theoretical frameworks available to inform relevant discussions in this area of public policy. This matters because recommendations about the need to support older workers will be restricted in the absence of theoretical models that shed light on factors that might limit their engagement in the labour market. In this context, there is a particular need for approaches that locate individual decision making both within life-course transitions as well as the broader political and economic institutions underpinning later life (Phillipson, 1998; Settersten and Trauten, 2009). Within sociology and social policy, relevant theoretical models include Bass and Caro's (2001) work in the field of productive ageing, Pillemer and colleagues' (2000) life-course approach to modelling retirement pathways, Sennett's (2006) analysis of the decline of 'work-based bureaucracies', and Phillipson's (1998) and Vickerstaff and Cox's (2005) work on the 'individualisation of retirement'. These approaches will be summarised to help contextualise empirical findings relating to training and education within and beyond employment.

The productive ageing approach has been the most explicit in theorising about obstacles to continued employment within the workplace, with a particular focus on examining evidence for discrimination or 'institutionalised ageism'. This model draws on 'cultural lag' theory (Riley and Riley, 1994) to explain the under-utilisation of older employees. The theory suggests that while retirement was originally premised on a surplus of labour, society may be slow to adapt workplace practices to the new reality of an ageing workforce and possible labour shortages. Bass and Caro (2001, p 56) argue that:

> With the rapid change in technology and the speed of innovation, individuals in virtually every profession and occupation are in need of lifelong learning. The current dominant life course pattern that emphasizes education when one is young, and heavy work demands in the early and middle career years ... may be incongruous with the pattern necessitated by a life course plan. Such a ... plan might be one where work demands are reduced in middle years and extended into the later years [or where there is] phased retirement.

Pillemer and colleagues' (2000) research reflects the importance of life-course perspectives in placing the experiences of older employees within a model that views the move from work to retirement as a process rather than a single or 'one-off' event. They extend this argument with the notion of 'linked lives' stretching across time and generations. Accordingly, 'retirement, family roles, community participation, and occupational careers are typically examined exclusive of other social roles and of each other. What we do not know is how work and family experiences shape life after retirement' (p 76). Or, to express this in a different way: *how do attitudes towards retirement or other social events shape experiences and approaches to working in later life?* What follows from this approach is that work and retirement can be seen as situated within a complex set of pathways in which biographical, health, occupational and economic factors interact, creating different degrees of attachment to paid employment.

The possibility of later life working will itself be influenced by a variety of organisational factors, not least the level of support provided within the work environment. Here, Ekerdt (2010, p 74) poses the question: '... *has the labor market become more welcoming to older workers, accommodating them in ways that could sustain an expansion in employment in later life*' (emphasis added). The evidence would suggest in fact only limited movement in practical steps to assist the extension of working life. Sennett (2006) argues that the collapse of the work-based bureaucracies associated with what he defines as 'social capitalism' has fostered a rise in 'precarious' and 'insecure employment' (to be discussed later). Social capitalism, it is argued, developed an 'ideal type' of work careers as long-term and incremental:

> Rationalized time enabled people to think about their lives as narratives — narratives not so much of what necessarily will happen as of how things should happen. It became possible, for instance, to define what the stages of a career ought to be like, to correlate long-term service in a firm to specific steps of increased wealth. (Sennett, 2006, p 23)

Sennett (2006, p 183) argued that the erosion of social capitalism 'deprived people of [a] sense of *narrative movement*' (emphasis in original). Elsewhere, he sets out a number of important questions that he sees as following from this development:

> How can long-term purposes be pursued in a short-term society? How can durable social relationships be sustained? How can a human being develop a narrative of identity and life history in a society composed of episodes and fragments? (Sennett, 1999, p 26)

In terms of the work-retirement transition, a number of research findings suggest the emergence of a more fragmented life-course. The expansion of so-called 'bridge jobs', along with the rise of self-employment, might be cited as one example, such employment becoming increasingly common for women and men in their 50s and 60s in the UK and US. Cahill and colleagues' (2006, p 523) research using data from the US Health and Retirement Study found that the majority of older Americans leaving full-time career employment (about 60% of those leaving a full-time career job after 50 and about 53% of those leaving after the age of 55) moved first to a bridge job rather than directly out of the labour force. Analysis of the British Household Panel Survey, examining job movements among men in their 50s, indicated that around one in five had spells of part-time, bridging forms of employment (Phillipson, 2002). Ekerdt (2010, p 75) makes the point that the characterisation of bridge jobs has important theoretical and ideological implications:

> Are older workers strategic, driven by values and goals, and able to control their conditions of work and the course of their late careers? Or, are they buffeted by structural changes at work that threaten their plans for an orderly and secure

retirement? One is an optimistic view of retirement, and one holds less cheer.

More generally, we can see 'bridging' and related forms of employment as part of the shift from the highly bureaucratised transition from work to retirement characteristic of the 1950s and 1960s, as contrasted with the more 'individualised', negotiated form that developed over the course of the 1990s (Phillipson, 1998; Vickerstaff and Cox, 2005). On the one hand, this development suggested a more agentic form of later life, with those moving from work to retirement 'richer, better educated and more culturally active ... than previous cohorts of retirees' (Gilleard and Higgs, 2005, p 14). On the other hand came evidence for increased inequality with scope for individual agency bounded or limited by the structural foundations associated with social class, gender, ethnic and employment location. Vickerstaff and Cox (2005, p 92) concluded that the consequence of individualisation for many older workers was '... less to increase the ... range of alternatives and choices over when and how to retire and more to enlarge the risks they had to cope with'.

Older workers, based on some of these accounts, would appear to have been affected by a variety of structural and organisational forces limiting choice and control within and beyond the workplace. In this context, moves to widen access to training and education for employment may be especially important. The next section of this chapter examines evidence for provision in this area, exploring developments over the course over the past two decades.

Training and education in the work and retirement transition

The benefit of training and learning, across all age groups, is now widely acknowledged. The Department for Education and Skills (DfES, 2005) argued that there was good evidence that 'older people can benefit substantially from continuing to learn and gain new skills' (para 210). Given a policy of extending the period of employment, the expectation must be that older workers will have an equal opportunity with younger age groups of sharing in different types of training and learning. The reality, however, based on a range of surveys in the UK and elsewhere, would suggest that this is invariably the exception rather than the rule. A benchmark survey of factors influencing older workers participation in employment by Humphrey and colleagues (2003) highlighted evidence for the sharp age-related decline in training. Of particular note was the extent to which encouragement from employers to learn new skills underwent a significant decline after age 55 – notably so in the case of men. Thus, over half of male employees (56%) reported little or no encouragement to learn more job-related skills compared with 44% of those aged 50-54; corresponding figures for women were 44% and 37%.

Lissenburgh and Smeaton's (2003) analysis of LFS data confirmed the link between increased age and declining access to training. Logistic regression models used in their study suggested that men and women in part-time and temporary employment were especially disadvantaged in respect of training. Humphrey and colleagues (2003) also found that the level of encouragement to undertake training varied between full- and part-time employees. In their survey, one third of part-time employees were offered no encouragement to learn more job-related skills, compared with one quarter of full-time employees. Such findings are especially important given the growth of 'non-standard' forms of work such as part-time and casual working, suggesting a likely increase over time in people denied access to training in the workplace.

Data from the LFS confirms the link between participation in training and socioeconomic status. Analysis of the 2008 survey found 35% of those in professional occupations having had training in the three months preceding the interview compared with 13% of those in routine occupations (Schuller and Watson, 2009). Occupational sector also appears to be influential: Schuller and Watson (2009, p 69) highlight the fact that working in the public sector gives a significant boost to accessing some form of training. Taking the proportion of people in employment age 25 to retirement who received some form of training in the three months prior to the interview, over 40% of public sector workers participated compared with 21% cent of those in the private sector. This is a highly significant contrast, given the projected decline in public sector employment, which has potentially serious consequences for access to training for older workers and other groups.

Newton and colleagues (2005) reported on the availability of training among those unemployed and economically inactive. This study shows that overall less than one in 10 report involvement in training and that training participation declines rapidly with age. The likelihood of someone aged 55 and over participating in training is 50% less compared with an adult aged 35-44. McNair and colleagues (2004) found that levels of support given to those changing their job declined with age. Older workers were less likely than younger ones to receive any help during a job transition (37% of older workers, against 47% of those under 50). They were less likely to receive training from their employers, help from their workmates and colleagues, or support from a government agency. They were also more likely to have sorted out support for themselves, either through the internet or other informal sources.

At the same time, it is important to recognise contradictory signs in the evidence for participation in training. Smeaton and colleagues (2010) make the point that many older workers remain committed to career development. In their survey, one third (33%) of 60- to 64-year-olds had undertaken training at some point in the previous three years. Cheung and Mckay (2010, p 38) noted some positive developments in participation trends, examining evidence from the LFS over the period 1994-2008. Although the researchers confirmed that training remained least common for the over-60s, participation had in fact increased over the period studied. The authors suggest that this: '... may be a positive sign that older workers are receiving opportunities that perhaps were [previously] more concentrated on younger workers'.

There is some evidence that workers may themselves show resistance to the idea of further training. This may happen where they lack confidence about learning new skills (Newton et al, 2003) or because they feel that acquiring them is unnecessary or may go unrewarded (McNair and Flynn, 2005). Taylor and Urwin's (2001) research conducted in the late 1990s suggested that declining participation in training was linked to employer decision making rather than individual preference not to undertake training. Urwin (2004, p 28), on the other hand, argues not only that is training less likely to be offered to older individuals, but also that 'large proportions of this group have not taken up the opportunity to train'. Information on this issue is provided by Felstead (2010) in research covering the employment experiences of workers in the UK aged 20-65. Findings from the 2006 Skills Survey used in the study indicated that around two thirds of men and women aged 50-65 said they 'did not want any training' compared with between one third and two fifths of younger workers. Older workers not in receipt of training also rated its benefits lower when compared with younger workers. Interestingly, the evidence did not point to employers being reluctant to provide training to older workers. Indeed, the reverse appeared to be the case, with a slightly higher proportion of younger workers reporting a lack of willingness on the part of their employer to provide training when it was wanted (Felstead, 2010, p 1310).

Employers are likely to vary considerably in their approach to training. McNair and colleagues (2004) found that people in large firms continued to develop skills in a way that was less true of those in small and medium-sized enterprises. Some groups – notably those drawn from managerial and professional backgrounds – appear much more likely to support training than others (for example, those in elementary occupations). Furthermore, level of skill and qualification (or human capital) appears critical – those with higher degrees and/or professional qualifications are more likely to participate in training later in working life compared with those with lower level qualifications (Newton et al, 2003). For professional/managerial groups, external pressure to extend working life may not be a major issue given that higher qualifications and socioeconomic class is a strong predictor of longer working life (McNair et al, 2004). For some manual groups, however, deficits in training over the life-course may be difficult to correct, especially given limited workplace opportunities and depressed expectations about learning (Schuller and Watson, 2009).

To these, largely negative, findings must be balanced more positive developments that may be important over the medium and longer term. Future generations of older workers can be expected to have higher levels of basic numeracy and literacy and this should have a major impact on participation in continuing education and training. Dixon (2003, p 74) notes from the LFS the strong relationship between level of qualification and the likelihood of undertaking job-related training, as well as the finding that those with higher existing qualifications are more likely to be studying for a new qualification. She concludes that: 'These relationships suggest that age-specific differentials in learning activity could flatten in future as the fraction of older workers who have not completed secondary education gradually declines'. On the other hand, stimulation and encouragement from employers and line managers will be vital if opportunities for training and learning are to be realised. The workplace remains a vital source for gaining knowledge about learning opportunities: 50% of people aged 45-54 found out about their current main learning activity through work (either their employer or workmates); the equivalent figure for those aged 55-64 was 30% (Aldridge and Tuckett, 2007). These figures will need to be built on, given a policy of extending working life, with a fresh emphasis on developing training and learning within the work environment. The next section of this chapter examines some key policies that will need to be developed.

Policy initiatives to expand training and education

The extent of change affecting work and retirement running through the period from the 1950s onwards suggests the need for innovation in what has become a key area for public policy. Among these, access to training and education in the second half of the life-course will be a crucial area for development, with significant implications for health and wellbeing in the workplace. Ford (2005a) makes the point that although many of those aged 50-60/65 possess skills and experience currently lost to the economy, learning requirements are higher than for younger age groups. One in three experiences literacy or numeracy problems, compared with one in five of those in their late 20s/early 30s. Mayhew and Rijkers (2004) stress the importance of 'continuous learning during the whole of working life as a means of reducing the dangers of labour market disadvantage in the older years' (p 14). Ford (2005b, p 10) makes the case for an 'overall national third age guidance and learning strategy, one which would be linked to the national skills strategy and which would enable adults from mid-life onwards to maximise their skills and potential' (see, further, Schuller and Watson, 2010). Assisting this process will, however, require a reversal of current policies that are reducing public funding for adult learners, with the greatest felt by those in the 50-plus age group (Aldridge and Tuckett, 2007).

Policies for change will need to focus on the following areas:

- developing entitlements for 'third-age learning';
- reassessing methodologies and techniques for training older workers;
- expanding provision for those in non-standard forms of employment; and
- developing the involvement of higher and further education.

The first of these has been addressed by Schuller and Watson (2009) as part of their inquiry into the future of lifelong learning. In their recommendations for change, they set out a four-stage model to encourage learning across the life-course, recognising different periods of development in the years up to 25, 25-50, 50-74 and 75-plus. They suggest that what has been termed the 'third age' (50-74) should be viewed as a central period for encouraging enhanced training and education opportunities, based on a more even distribution of work across the life-course. This would be buttressed by a fairer allocation of educational resources (public, private and employer-based) to meet the needs of third- and fourth-age (those aged 75 plus) groups; a legal entitlement of free access to learning to acquire basic skills (for example, in literacy and numeracy); a 'good practice' entitlement to learning leave as an occupational benefit; and specific 'transition entitlements', for example for people on their 50th birthday, to 'signal the continuing potential for learning of those moving into the third age' (Schuller and Watson, 2009, p 133).

The second area raises issues about developing more effective training programmes targeted at older adults. The research evidence reviewed earlier suggests that employer (or line manager) 'discouragement' partly explains decreasing participation in training. Yet it is also clear that this not a complete explanation for the problem. In particular, workers themselves may consider – after a certain age or stage in their career – that further training is unnecessary, or they may feel that the type of training and learning they are likely to receive is inappropriate given their level of skill and experience. Czaja and Sharit (2009, p 266) make the point that although many existing training techniques are effective for older adults, we lack an adequate research database to '… determine whether some training techniques are consistently differentially beneficial to older workers'. On the other hand, literature from work-based psychological studies has demonstrated the benefits as well as limitations of particular approaches to training involving older workers. Tsang (2009, p 289), for example, cites a number of studies that show how relatively small amounts of training can reverse cognitive decline and assist the retention of newly acquired skills. Conversely, the limitations of training benefits are also noted, including reduced magnitude of learning and slower learning rates. Given the emergence of a more diverse ageing workforce, attention to new ways of delivering work-based training would seem an urgent requirement. One suggestion here would be to encourage a single organisation to lead research and policy initiatives linking trades unions, business organisations and government around the theme of training for an ageing workforce. This would require dedicated funding and staffing, but could be part of an existing body (the Third Age Employment Network would be one organisation that could take the lead in developing such an initiative).

The third area concerns the need to encourage training programmes specifically targeted at those in part-time and flexible forms of employment, and with those older workers who are self-employed. The issues here have been summarised by Czaja and Sharit (2009, p 259) as follows:

> … as the number of workers in non-standard work arrangements … continues to increase, one important issue confronting workers will be access to traditional workplace benefits such as training. [Such] workers will be less likely to receive structured company-sponsored training and the responsibility of continuous learning and job training will fall to a greater extent on the individual. It is not yet clear

how to best develop and disseminate training programs to promote lifelong learning for these 'non-traditional' workers. This issue is especially pertinent for older workers, given that they are less likely to be provided with access to training and development programmes in traditional work environments where company-sponsored training is available.

There are no easy solutions to the problems facing part-time and related groups of workers. On the one hand, studies cited earlier (for example, Humphrey et al, 2003; Lissenburgh and Smeaton, 2003) highlight inequalities between full- and part-time workers in respect of access to training. Such difficulties are unlikely to have changed – they have probably worsened – in the period since the research was published. On the other hand, opportunities from providers such as community and further education colleges have been steadily reduced, with the major focus now placed on preparing younger people for entry into the labour market. Some options for consideration here might include, first, adoption of Schuller and Watson's (2009) plan for legal and transitional entitlements (mentioned earlier), a proposal highly relevant to those entering non-standard and flexible forms of employment; second, more imaginative use of computer-based training or 'e-learning' to assist those working from home or those juggling work and care-giving responsibilities (Czaja and Sharit, 2009); and third, specific obligations placed on employers to expand training and learning as a precondition for creating non-standard forms of employment.

The final area for discussion concerns encouraging closer involvement from higher and further education in responding to the needs of older workers, with the development of new programmes or the adaptation of existing courses. Older students have always had an important presence in university adult education classes, with those over 50 comprising the majority of participants. They also form a significant group studying for part-time degrees and programmes related to continuing professional development (Phillipson, 2010). The number of older learners moving into higher education will almost certainly increase, given broader demographic and social changes. Key factors are likely to include, first, the demand for vocational and non-vocational courses coming from 'first-wave' baby boomers (those born in the late-1940s and early-1950s), a larger proportion of whom – in comparison with earlier cohorts – have degrees and related qualifications; and second, the need for new qualifications among those changing careers in mid- and later working life. Reflecting this development, three pathways might be followed by higher education institutions to support older workers:

- *Educational and personal development programmes*: these would build on existing work in adult and continuing education, but would identify new types of courses and markets among a diverse and segmented post-50s market.
- *Employment-related programmes*: these might support the policy objective of extending working life, although the extent of employer demand may be fragile in the context of high levels of unemployment. The development of courses supporting people moving from full-time paid employment to various forms of self-employment may, however, remain a source of growth among higher education institutions (HEIs).
- *Social inclusion programmes*: substantial numbers of older people – in current as well as succeeding cohorts – remain educationally and socially disadvantaged. HEIs, with partners such as local authorities, further education colleges and the major national charities, should focus on a 'widening participation' agenda that covers all age groups and not just younger adults.

Conclusion

Demands to extend working life inevitably raise issues about the training available to assist career and skill development in the workplace. To date, those entering the later stages of their careers are unlikely to be encouraged to learn new or optimise existing skills. Even where this is the case, doubts may persist about the value or quality of training on offer. Of equal concern is the fact that those sectors where training is emphasised (such as the public sector) are in decline, while areas undergoing expansion (such as part-time working) often provide low-level and poor-quality training. From a policy perspective, three issues will need to be considered as a part of a strategy for training to support an extended working life. First, encouraging lifelong learning – especially among those with limited skills and poor educational attainment – remains a priority. In the absence of a firm commitment to improve training and education for older workers, greater inequality – in work experiences and expectations – is inevitable. Second, research is needed to examine the benefits of training and professional development, not just for the acquisition of new skills but for the promotion of health and wellbeing more generally. With budgets for training under inevitable pressure, demonstrating what works, for whom, and in what way, will be increasingly important.

Third, innovative projects will be required to meet the training and educational needs of a group comprising age cohorts with contrasting educational and social backgrounds. Rethinking the nature of training provision is a key requirement if an extending working life is to be realised. Fourth, recognising the complexity of the work-retirement transition remains important. Workers will continue to 'anticipate their retirement' even while maintaining or extending their working life. Recognising the linkages between employment and retirement will be a significant element in human resource strategies for the 21st century.

Further reading

Czaja, S. and Sharit, J. (eds) (2009) *Aging and work: Issues and implications in a changing landscape*, Baltimore, NJ: The John Hopkins University Press.

DWP (Department for Work and Pensions) (2009) *Building a society for all ages*, London: DWP.

Ekerdt, D. (2010) 'Frontiers of research on work and retirement', *The Gerontologist*, vol 65b, no 1, pp 69-80.

Phillipson, C. and Ogg, J. (2010) *Active ageing and universities: Engaging older learners*, London: Universities UK.

Schuller, T. and Watson, D. (2009) *Learning through life*, Leicester: National Institute of Adult and Continuing Education.

References

Aldridge, F. and Tuckett, A. (2007) *What older people learn*, Leicester: National Institute of Adult and Continuing Education.

Bass, S.A. and Caro, F.G. (2001) 'Productive aging: a conceptual framework', in N. Morrow-Howell, J. Hinterland and M. Sherraden (eds) *Productive aging*, Baltimore, NJ: The John Hopkins University Press, pp 37-80.

Cahill, K., Giandrea, M and Quinn, J. (2006) 'Retirement patterns from career employment', *The Gerontologist*, vol 46, no 4, pp 514-23.

Cheung, S. and McKay, S. (2010) *Training and progression in the labour market*, Research Report No 680, London: Department for Work and Pensions.

Czaja, S. and Sharit, J. (2009) 'Preparing organizations and older workers for current and future employment', in S.J. Czaja and J. Sharit (eds) *Aging and work: Issues and implications in a changing landscape*, Baltimore, NJ: The John Hopkins University Press, pp 259-78.

DfES (Department for Education and Skills) (2005) *Skills: Getting on in business, getting on in work. Parts 1-3*, London: The Stationery Office.

Dixon, S (2003) 'Implications of population ageing for the labour market', *Labour Market Trends*, vol 111, no 2, pp 67-76.

DWP (Department for Work and Pensions) (2005) *Opportunity age*, London: HMSO.

Ekerdt, D. (2010) 'Frontiers of research on work and retirement'. *The Gerontologist*, vol 65b, no 1, pp 69-80.

EHRC (Equality and Human Rights Commission) (2010) *Working better: The over 50s, the new work generation*, London: EHRC.

Felstead, A. (2010) 'Closing the age gap? Age, skills and the experience of work in Great Britain' *Ageing & Society*, 30, pp 1293-314.

Ford, G. (2005a) *Am I still needed? Guidance and learning for older adults*, Derby: University of Derby, Centre for Guidance Studies.

Ford, G. (2005b) 'Am I still needed? Guidance and learning for older adults', in D. Hirsch (ed) *Sustaining working lives: A framework for policy and practice*, York: Joseph Rowntree Foundation.

Giddens, A. (1991) *Modernity and self-identity*, Cambridge: Polity Press.

Gilleard, C. and Higgs, P. (2005) *Contexts of ageing*, Cambridge: Polity Press.

Humphrey, A., Costigan, P., Pickering, K., Stratford, N. and Barnes, M. (2003) *Factors affecting the labour market: Participation of older workers*, London: Department for Work and Pensions

Laczko, F. and Phillipson, C. (1991) *Changing work and retirement*, Maidenhead: Open University Press.

Lissenburgh, S. and Smeaton, D. (2003) *Employment transitions of older workers: The role of flexible employment in maintaining labour market participation and promoting job quality*, Bristol and York: Policy Press and Joseph Rowntree Foundation.

Marshall, V.W., Heinz, W.R., Krüger, H. and Vermer, A. (eds) (2001) *Restructuring work and the life course*, Toronto: University of Toronto Press.

McNair, S. and Flynn, M. (2005) *The age dimension of employment practice: Employer case studies*, London: Department of Trade and Industry.

McNair, S., Flynn, M., Owen, L., Humphreys, C. and Woodfield, S. (2004) *Changing work in later life: A study of job transitions*, Guildford: University of Surrey, Centre for Research into the Older Workforce.

Mayhew, K. and Rijkers, B. (2004) 'How to improve the human capital of older workers, or the sad tail of the magic bullet', Paper presented to the joint EC–OECD seminar on Human Capital and Labour Market Performance, Brussels, 8 December.

Newton, B., Hirshfield, J., Miller, L., Ackroyd, K. and Gifford, J. (2003) *Training participation amongst unemployed and inactive people*, Brighton: Institute for Employment Studies.

Newton, B., Hirschfield, J., Miller, L. and Bates, P. (2005) *Training a mixed age workforce: Practical tips and guidance*, London: Department for Work and Pensions.

OECD (Organisation for Economic Co-operation and Development) (2006) *Live longer, work longer*, Paris, OECD.

Pensions Commission (2004) *Pensions: Challenges and choices*, Norwich: The First Report of the Pensions Commission, London: The Stationery Office.

Phillipson, C. (1993) 'The sociology of retirement', in J. Bond, P. Coleman and S. Peace (eds) *Ageing and society: An introduction to social gerontology*, London: Sage Publications.

Phillipson, C. (1998) *Reconstructing old age: New agendas in social theory and social practice*, London: Sage Publications.

Phillipson, C. (2002) *Transitions from work to retirement: New patterns of work and retirement*, Bristol: The Policy Press.

Phillipson, C. (2009) 'Pensions in crisis: aging and inequality in a global age', in L. Rogne, C. Estes, B. Grossman, B. Hollister and E. Solway (eds) *Social insurance and social justice*, New York, NY: Springer Publishing.

Phillipson, C. (2010) 'Active ageing and universities: engaging older learners', *International Journal of Education and Ageing*, vol 1, no 1, pp 9-22.

Phillipson, C. and Smith, C. (2005) *Extending working life: A review of the research literature*, London: Department for Work and Pensions.

Pillemer, K., Moen, P., Wethington, E. and Glasgow N. (eds) (2000) *Social integration in the second half of life*, Baltimore, NJ: John Hopkins University Press.

PIU (Performance and Innovation Unit) (2000) *Winning the generation game*, London: The Stationery Office.

Riley, M. and Riley, J.W. Jnr (1994) 'Structural lag: past and future', in M. Riley, R. Kahn, and A. Foner (eds) *Age and structural lag*, New York, NY: John Wiley & Sons, pp 15-36.

Schuller, T. and Watson, D. (2009) *Learning through life: Inquiry into the Future for Lifelong Learning*, Leicester: National Institute of Adult and Continuing Education.

Sennett, R. (1999) *The corrosion of character*, New York, NY: W.W. Norton.

Sennett, R. (2006) *The culture of the new capitalism*, New Haven, CT: Yale University Press.

Settersten, R. and Trauten, M. (2009) 'The new terrain of old age: hallmarks, freedoms and risks', in V. Bengston, D. Gans, N. Putney and M. Silverstein (eds) *Handbook of theories of aging*, New York, NY: Springer, pp 455-70.

Smeaton, D., Vegaris, S. and Sahin-Dikmen, M. (2010) *Older workers: Employment preferences, barriers and solutions*, London: Policy Studies Institute.

Taylor, P. and Urwin, P. (2001) 'Age and participation in vocational education and training', *Work, Employment and Society*, vol 15, pp 763-79.

TAEN (Third Age Employment Network) (2011) *Newsletter New Year 2011*, London: TAEN.

Tsang, T. (2009) 'Age and performance measures of knowledge-based work: a cognitive perspective', in S.J. Czaja and J. Sharit (eds) *Aging and work: Issues and implications in a changing landscape*, Baltimore, NJ: John Hopkins University Press, pp 279-306.

Urwin, P. (2004) *Age matters: A review of existing survey evidence*, Employment Relations Research Series No 24, London: Department of Trade and Industry.

Vickerstaff, S. and Cox, J. (2005) 'Retirement and risk: the individualisation of retirement and experiences?', *The Sociological Review*, vol 53, pp 77-95.

Vickerstaff, S. (2010) 'Older workers: the "unavoidable obligation" of extending our working lives?', *Sociology Compass*, vol 4, no 10, pp 869-79.

FOURTEEN

Conclusion: setting the agenda for future research

Chris Phillipson, Ross Wilkie and Sarah Vickerstaff

The first decade of the 21st century saw a profound shift in perspectives on the nature of work across the life-course. For much of the preceding five decades, there was a steady redistribution of activity from work to retirement. In 1950, the average age of exit (for men) from employment was 67.2 years, with life expectancy of 10.8 years at age of exit from the workforce; by 2004, estimates from the Pensions Commission indicated that the average age of exit from work had dropped to 63.8 years, with a near doubling of life expectancy after exit from employment to 20.1 years (Pensions Commission, 2004). More recently, however, this shift in the allocation of time has come under scrutiny, with ageing populations and their perceived costs raising demands to extend working life (IPSPC, 2011; OECD, 2011; see, further, Chapter One of this volume). Yet, as the various contributors to this collection demonstrate, achieving this will require intervention across the various stages of people's working lives. This raises a substantial set of tasks for employers, employees, trades unions and government. Managing health in the workplace, and securing the wellbeing of employees, has to be a central goal if extension of working life is to be realised. Given this context, the purpose of this book has been to place on the agenda the range of issues that an effective 'health in the workplace' policy will need to achieve. Clearly, the variety of topics is extensive, covering as a minimum the nature of work, workplace design, organisational power and dynamics, mental and physical health, work incapacity, vocational rehabilitation, and education and training. Such a list provides a significant agenda for researchers and policy organisations concerned both with extending and promoting the quality of working life.

The purpose of this final chapter is to draw together some of the research issues identified in the preceding chapters. These can be used to provide a basis for setting out the key tasks that need to be addressed if a healthier working life is to be achieved. Drawing on the various recommendations from the authors in this book, we identify five major areas for research:

- increasing our understanding of different types of organisation;
- improving the work environment;
- developing effective interventions;
- developing a user perspective; and
- securing effective multidisciplinary/multicentre studies.

These areas will each be discussed in turn followed by a summary of the main arguments.

Increasing our understanding of different organisations

Virtually all the chapters in this book have highlighted the significance of the organisational context for understanding issues relating to work and wellbeing. From a research perspective, however, a number of contributors note the extent to which much of our knowledge has been shaped by work in large organisations, neglecting the fact that small and medium-sized enterprises (SMEs) provide the location for the majority of employees. Yet SMEs, as Fehmidah Munir notes in Chapter Eleven, may often lack the resources to provide an integrated response to assist health promotion in the workplace, one that draws on the full range of professionals available to provide advice and support. Annie Irvine, also in the context of SMEs, highlights in Chapter Three the need for better understanding of mental health issues, noting their impact on co-workers as well as the productivity of firms. The case for researching the influence of organisations on heath and wellbeing is made by Julia Gibbs and colleagues in Chapter Twelve, notably in the context of organisational change in the NHS. But the research evidence about the role of organisations in promoting or restricting health and wellbeing remains limited and focused around particular types of (invariably large) organisations. In consequence, we need to research more detailed questions such as:

- Who are the groups most affected by organisational change?
- What specific consequences for mental and physical health can be identified?
- What variations are there across different types of organisation?
- Can we identify specific types of responses – resilience, resistance or passivity – that individuals develop to guard against the pressures raised by organisational change?

A further element in a future research agenda must be more detailed consideration of the role of line managers in supporting workers experiencing mental and physical health problems. Line managers (LMs) play a crucial role (whether directly or indirectly) in managing health issues, just as they will influence decision making about whether individuals remain in employment up to and beyond state pension age. But although the importance of line managers is well established, we know very little about the nature of the role they play when support – both short- and long-term – is required. Again, some important questions here might include: How do LMs vary in the kind of assistance offered to workers? To what extent is any variation linked to differences in organisational context? Is the knowledge base of LMs adequate for supporting workers with health problems? What types of intervention, including training programmes, might be developed to increase their influence in securing positive outcomes for those with health problems?

Improving the work environment

Many of the chapters in this book provide a specific challenge in arguing that the work environment itself may be culpable in promoting higher levels of stress and disability. This is not to argue against views about the benefits of work as a force assisting the integration of individuals into society (see, for example, Black, 2008). Rather, the point (as made by Annie Irvine in Chapter Three; see also Chapter One) is that in the context of health and wellbeing 'good work may be good' but 'bad work' may indeed be harmful. The issues raised by various contributors suggest a number of research questions that require attention. A starting point would be to examine whether workplace conditions have deteriorated to the extent of being a threat to good health, and, if this is the case, to which groups this might apply. Certainly, there appears the possibility for this, especially given the rise of part-time employment and increased levels of job insecurity, both of which are linked to some of the economic and social risks posed by globalisation. All of this raises the need for more research about the impact of work on the individual, a pressing need in the context of pressures to extend working life. Some questions here include: Will prolonged work enhance or reduce wellbeing for certain groups? If the former, are there lessons that can be applied across work environments more generally? If the latter, what different types of interventions can be devised to reduce the problems experienced across different points of the life-course? How can employees – across all age groups – gain more power to influence the quality of the working environment? A particular need here is for longitudinal research able to test out new approaches to improving working life and in particular the value of models such as that of 'work ability' discussed in the chapter by Tony Maltby in Chapter Ten.

At the same time, as some of the contributors also note, there is a strong subjective component in responses to pressures at work. Julia Gibbs and colleagues in Chapter Twelve make the point that employees may be more accurately viewed as 'active agents' in shaping changes to their working lives. In Chapter Nine, David Wainwright and Michael Calnan build on this argument in viewing 'the lived experience of the worker' as a mediating element between 'objective' work conditions and 'subjective' experiences. From a research perspective, better understanding is needed of the balance between such 'objective' and 'subjective' factors in determining responses to particular types of workplace problems. The implication of some of the chapters (for example, Chapters Four and Seven) is that certain groups – such as those on low incomes or those living in a geographical context of weak labour markets – may find 'actively shaping' responses to health difficulties a considerable challenge. In contrast, better understanding is needed of the strategies adopted by some groups to maintain control of their work environments, alongside the associated benefits for managing changes in physical and mental health. The important issue here is that while many of the issues facing people at work may have common causes and origins, the reactions to these will be as varied as the biographies and circumstances of the individuals affected. This observation underlines David Wainwright and colleagues' argument about the need for an 'individualised' approach to managing people's re-entry into work – a point that may also be extended to the broader range of issues people face within the workplace. Moreover, variation in approach will be especially pronounced, given the diversity of social networks and social support available to individuals. In this context, health promotion at work must of necessity extend beyond addressing particular circumstances and relationships within employment, and also consider the role of family, friends and other aspects of community support. An issue for the research agenda concerns the need to consider the full range of relationships within which individuals are embedded, assessing the particular contribution each makes to physical and/or mental health issues. A research focus on the social context influencing the individual would provide a more robust account of the effects of the social in biopsychosocial models of ill health.

Developing effective interventions

The range and complexity of issues facing people within the workplace has been a prominent theme of this book. In this regard, a common concern running through many of the chapters is the lack of good-quality evidence about *'what works best'*, *'for whom'* and for *'what type of condition'*. In Chapter Two, Ross Wilkie identifies some of the problems here when discussing the extent (and complexity) of co-morbidity, for example, musculoskeletal conditions linked to mental health problems such as depression. He emphasises the importance (along with Tony Maltby and others) of a 'biopsychosocial approach' to managing health issues, with interventions directed towards a more 'proactive preventive health model'. In Chapter Three, Annie Irvine highlights the limited evidence base in respect of understanding interventions that can help people cope with common mental health problems at work. In Chapter Eight, David Wainwright and colleagues further make the point that in the absence of strong evidence, 'off-the-shelf', and in consequence often ineffective, interventions are much more likely.

The first stage in developing effective interventions must be to address the still limited understanding about the impact of health problems within the workplace. Lack of detailed information is still leading to off-the-shelf interventions focusing on single issues rather than the combination of conditions affecting people in middle and older age. Moreover, the role of co-morbidity and its cumulative effect highlights the need to conduct longitudinal research, rather than focus on cross-sectional findings, to clearly outline cause and effect. As highlighted throughout this book, a life-course approach would also be beneficial, particular to achieving prevention. To develop effective interventions, older workers must become a greater focus for research, given the emphasis now placed on the extending working-life agenda. The next step must be to identify groups of older workers who are at risk of particular problems and who may be especially receptive to certain types of interventions. Off-the-shelf interventions could be a starting point, but evaluation of why they are successful or unsuccessful is important for further development. Developing methodologies in both epidemiological studies and trials is important to the process.

The Pathways to Work and Fit for Work Services pilots provide examples of the type of interventions that may enhance health and work. In addition to managing health issues (single conditions and co-morbidity), the link with employers and employment systems is a positive approach to enhancing work participation. Again, appropriate evaluation is important for further evolution of interventions and these pilots should be seen as a starting point rather than one that provides a definitive approach.

Developing a user perspective

Identifying how users themselves view the different support services is itself a vital area for research. David Wainwright and colleagues make the case here for qualitative studies that can provide policymakers and service providers with an 'in-depth understanding' of how users experience service uptake and how interventions 'affect their sense of self and identity'. This clearly highlights the role that the user's perspective has in research, helping to identify and prioritise areas for research and potential targets to reduce health and work problems. Systematic evidence about user views is also clearly essential, along with quantitative research, for the development of effective interventions within the workplace. Yet this area remains underdeveloped in at least three main respects:

First, user-related research needs to draw in a wider range of groups than is presently the case. We might include here those in part-time employment – especially minority ethnic groups such as South Asian groups (for example, Bangladeshis and Pakistanis) where chronic health problems sit alongside low-wage/low-skill employment, and those in particular employment sectors (for example, agriculture) where ill health in mid-life may be especially damaging for prospects of continued employment.

Second, the methodological approaches for involving users require clarification and development. Qualitative methods are typically cited as the best approach, but refinement of the best and most appropriate techniques is necessary. More work is required on the problems of gaining user views in contexts where employees (as well as employers) may be suspicious of the value of research – and the ends to which it is put. This may become a particular problem in a sustained period of economic recession where individuals may be more concerned with 'hiding' rather than 'disclosing' workplace problems.

Third, some broadening in the range of groups defined as users is also required. Employers are clearly of considerable importance, but carers also need similar acknowledgement as supporters in many cases to people with workplace problems. Ensuring that different groups are given 'equal voice' in the user research process is crucial and suggests the need for a number of demonstration projects to indicate the benefits of this approach.

It is also worth noting the strength of including the user's perspective and of users' active involvement in conducting research, with input to methodological development, interpretation of results and dissemination. Users are able to comment on the design and feasibility of projects in real-life environments and add to the experience and expertise of the research group. This was evident during network meetings (the origins of this book; see Chapter One) when users were able to comment on whether suggested methods to explore an intervention to change the behaviour of line managers would be possible in particular work environments. This builds on the role of users' involvement in face validity studies to ensure the acceptability and comprehensibility of measurement tools (such as questionnaires). At a later stage, perhaps in the form of advisory groups, user input is constructive and ensures a comprehensive approach to the interpretation of findings. Dissemination by users ensures greater implementation of findings. Employers and agencies (for example, the Department for Work and Pensions) may implement findings quickly. Patient and public involvement conferences provide further opportunities for dissemination and development of user input. User-led research is encouraged and provides a further opportunity to enhance our understanding of the health and work process.

Securing effective multidisciplinary/multicentre studies

Two of the recurrent themes in this book are first, that the relationship between work and health is a complex phenomenon and, second, that a multidimensional approach is required to understand it. Interaction, including acceptance of different approaches and views, between a range of disciplines focusing on health and work will broaden the knowledge base and understanding of health and work. This joined-up approach will maximise the benefits of improving health in the workplace. Individual disciplines have a detailed understanding of some factors that affect health and work: for example, epidemiologists in relation to the impact of musculoskeletal conditions; occupational psychologists in relation to workplace stress. A collaborative approach would:

- enable better understanding of the interactions between the various factors affecting health in the workplace;
- enhance the development of new research questions and opportunities;
- drive the development of novel research approaches to manage the complexities of work and health in older adults;

- lead to further creation of new collaborations between researchers, employers, government agencies, the third sector and employees, all focused on maximising improvement in health and work for older workers.

To achieve this, research teams should combine expertise in qualitative and quantitative methods, from both clinicians and non-clinicians, together with disciplines such as epidemiology, occupational psychology and sociology. Research teams should aim to maximise the translation of their work into policy and practice and develop further collaborative research by working alongside stakeholders. The formation of research centres focusing on the topic is one way forward. It is possible that greater gains might be made by multicentre collaborations to enable combined working between national and international leaders and the pulling together of state-of-the-art methodologies and findings to drive knowledge and research.

Conclusion

Working life is likely to undergo a number of major changes in the 21st century. In the case of industrialised economies, the dominant trends are likely to be a continued shift from manufacturing to the service sector, a rise in part-time and self-employment, and pressure on individuals to continue to work into their 60s and 70s. At the same time, there is evidence of rising levels of insecurity in the workplace, high levels of unemployment (especially among young people but increasingly among women as well) and problems of underemployment and deskilling. Resolving these tensions will be vital for maintaining health and wellbeing in the workplace. Comprehensive strategies will be required to secure effective support for those experiencing physical and mental ill health in middle and later working life, those seeking to re-enter work after an extended period of unemployment and those planning to continue to work into their late 60s and beyond. Such strategies will need to be sensitive to the different groups requiring support – for example, those from different ethnic groups and those experiencing co-morbid conditions – as well as being alert to the needs of those providing help within the workplace. This book has set out some of the issues that will need to be tackled by government, employers, trades unions and workers themselves, in the years ahead. We hope that it provides a useful stimulus to debate and policy development in a major area of social and public policy.

References

Black, C. (2008) *Working for a healthier tomorrow*, London: The Stationery Office.

IPSPC (Independent Public Service Pensions Commission) (2011) *Final report*, London: IPSPC.

OECD (Organisation for Economic Co-operation and Development) (2011) *Pensions at a glance 2011: Retirement income systems in OECD and G20 countries*, Paris: OECD.

Pensions Commission (2004) *Pensions: Challenges and choices*, Norwich: The First Report of the Pensions Commission, London: The Stationery Office.

Index

The letter f following a page note indicates a figure, n and endnote and t a table